LET ME GET THIS OFF MY CHEST

*An inspiring story of saving my own
life and my journey to self-love*

Tara Hopko

Published by T & MH Services

Printing in the United States of America
First printing 2019

ISBN: 9781791826963

To Matt, Maddie, Lexie & Mama Lu

Thank you for your love and support through the most difficult journey of my life. Thank you for picking me up when I was down, for always believing in me, and loving me even when I didn't love myself.

To My Amazing Friends

Thank you for being there on the ugly days and reminding me that I am stronger than I could ever imagine.

To My Sister-in-Law ~ Valerie

Thank you for blessing me with your time and talent editing my work.

To Cortney Torres Photography

Thank you for your amazing skills and being part of this 'chapter' in my journey.

Cover Design Credit:
To the extraordinary Valerie Gyorgy,
valerie@re-think.ca

To Dr. Brian Buinewicz, MD:

Thank you for your kind spirit, your gentle understanding and most of all, for saving my life.

To Dr. Alex Mercado, MD:

Thank you for never telling me I was crazy and for your relentless efforts in attempting to help me with my endless symptoms.

To Elaine Hardy:

You are a gift. Your knowledge and beautiful spirit inspired me to never give up the search for what was ailing me. Thank you for being so generous and always believing in me.

To my Fellow BII sisters:

This book is dedicated to all of you. We are warriors and are not fighting this battle alone. May you always see the beauty that lies within you and know you are always enough just as God created you.

CONTENTS

~ INTRODUCTION ~

Is this me? How did I get here? Crumbled in the fetal position on the shower floor, head in my hands, quietly sobbing. You have to be quiet, I think to myself. You can't let them know the kind of pain you are in. All I can think is, I don't even want my children to know this kind of pain exists, let alone that their mother is silently dying on the inside. Pull yourself together, I whisper. I'm convulsing- the kind of crying you feel in your soul, the kind that leaves you with nothing left on the inside once the storm has passed. I can't seem to pull myself out of this. The tears keep coming. I want to scream, but all I can do is align my face with the shower stream to assure I won't make a sound.

As the water pelts my face, my husband and our two daughters are busy in the rooms across the hall. They cannot know this is happening, I'm not ready to justify this level of sadness to anyone quite yet. I'm not even sure what's happening to me; so how the hell could I explain this to someone, especially my most loved ones. This experience is similar to those times in my teens when I was sad and hopeless, sitting on the roof of my house hanging on for dear life, but praying to fall off at the same time. But you expect that from a raging hormonal teenage girl.

This was unexpected; this was a levelheaded working mother who appeared to have it all together. Things like this didn't happen to level headed working moms... or did they? Was that it? Was it like the doctors have been saying? I'm just stressed, overworked, and tired. My instincts told me, NO. This wasn't a normal breakdown of a busy, overtired mom. There was more to what was happening here, but what? And how will I find out what's happening if I can't even muster up the strength to get off the floor of the shower?

These reminiscent thoughts of my teen years and these questions in my mind appear to slap me back into reality. The convulsing has begun to subside. I manage to pull myself off the floor into an upright position. I'm dizzy and I'm not sure if it's due to all the crying or that I've been lying in a hot shower for what seemed like hours. *Deep breaths*, I think to myself, *if you could just take some deep breaths you'll feel better.* However, I don't feel better, I can't take a deep breath. I can't even seem to catch my breath at all for that matter. Again, it could be due to the hot steamy shower, but everything in my gut tells me, that's not it.

My breath has escaped me for a long while now and that's just a small part of what's been going on lately. For the past few years my brain resembles the current state of the mirror in my shower, completely fogged. Nothing has been clear to me in a very long time. Not until now that is. My ah-ha moment finally occurs, right here in the heat of my bathroom, while I silently sob to myself. For the first time in a long time, I finally have a thought of clarity. Something is seriously wrong with me and although the doctors seem to think this is all "perfectly normal", I am no longer taking that as an answer! I will pull myself together and take my life back from whatever this is that's eating me alive, or I'll die trying. In that moment there was one thing I knew for sure; I could no longer live like this but I didn't want to die.

I turned the water off, amazed there was any left after my extended stay and as I grabbed the towel to wipe my swollen eyes, there was a knock at the door. "You OK in there?" My husband asked. "The girls and I are ready to start the movie, we are just waiting on you." "Yes, I am OK," I lied. "I'll be right out." Thankful, he was innocently clueless enough to not realize the truth behind my lie. There was nothing OK about me anymore. There hadn't been for a long time. But why? How did I get here? What the hell is wrong with me? I crept

3

down the stairs and met my family with a painted smile on my face keeping my head down, assuring no 'swollen' eye contact is made as I've done so many times before. "I'm ready," I say.

Chapter One
~ How Did I Get Here ~

Long before I ended up in the fetal position on my shower floor at 38 years old, I was a pretty normal girl. I grew up in New Jersey in a family of four, which eventually turned into divorced families of two and two but that was not front-page news in the 90's. There were issues and the kind of scars you can't see, but those are pages for a different book. I had all the support I needed growing up, even when it was just my mom and I. She was a woman of much strength and lots of independence. Growing up just the two of us gave me a lot of character and appreciation for the little things in life. The hidden scars left behind could have led me down the wrong path several times in my life, but I was saved. Saved by the first love in my life. Dancing.

As a competitive dancer, I was able to transform into someone else on stage, anyone I wanted to be. The multiple practices during the week and on weekends assured my mom I would not get into trouble. Dancers are tough on themselves. Always trying to be better, faster, and stronger than the next girl. And skinny. When you're tossing yourself in the air it pays to be thin, especially while doing it in a leotard and tights. I had many friends in my dance years, and as we matured it became harder and harder to remain without the noticeable curves of a typical 17-year-old girl. Extreme measures were taken sometimes. Not just eating the cookies at break time, but tossing them immediately afterward in the toilet in hopes the calories wouldn't count. After several years of watching numerous friends suffer through bulimia and anorexia, I became grateful for escaping the disorders.

Having curves that dancers typically didn't have, I would desperately attempt to 'tuck my butt' at my ballet teacher's request but God did not intend for my ass to do anything but project outward. I embraced it and my boyfriend didn't seem to mind that 'baby got back' so why not, right? Now, although my lower region was rich in the curves department, my upper half seemed to be lacking. Contrary to my mother's belief, and thanks to a misleading early development, I was not the "big chested" girl she was worried I would be. In fact, as I stood in the dance studio getting fitted for our costumes, I would marvel at the likes of the other girls who had boobs. Envious of the fact they had to tape their breasts down to make them less noticeable in their costume, I pondered if I even needed a bra at all.

Although my dance teachers were thrilled I was a member of the itty-bitty titty committee, I began to feel less of a woman with small boobs. After all, society has shoved big boobs in our faces for a long time. We are figuratively motor-boated by magazines, commercials and advertisements constantly. Everywhere you turn there are women flaunting their well-endowed chests. To say I felt left out was an understatement. Nevertheless, I didn't let my small boobs get me down in those days. In fact, I was full of life growing up and especially while dancing on stage. I enjoyed every bit of being the center of attention.

At one of my most memorable competitions, I had just performed the heck out of a lyrical dance routine, *Via Dolorosa*. It was an emotional piece where I portrayed the figure of Mary while walking alongside Jesus on the way to his crucifixion. I felt every moment of that dance to my core, leaping and spinning, covering the entire stage with my emotions. As the routine ended, my whole body was trembling with my dramatic interpretation of how it must have felt to watch your blood die on the cross. At the end of the award ceremony that day, the judges gave out special awards for different outstanding performances. That night, I walked away with the "Most Likely to Become an Actress" award. I was thrilled with this honor, the judges recognizing my passion for transforming into someone else up on that stage.

In the eleven years I danced competitively, I lived for those three-minute clips of time under the lights. Never once did I think twice about how I looked in my costumes up on stage. I was never a self-conscious person; in fact, I prided myself on my confidence. When I was entering puberty, my dance teachers thought I would be one of the 'bigger' girls. In reality, I never really grew much at all after sixth grade. So, by my last year of dance at eighteen years old, I was never the tallest or the thinnest, but I prided myself on having a hell of a lot of heart.

In my teens I felt there was hope in regards to the small chest issue. "After you have kids you'll develop bigger boobs," my mom would tell me. As I entered adulthood, her words were always in the back of my mind. Big boobs after kids made sense and if I could score anything larger than my current small B cup, I would be thrilled.

In 2004, I married my best friend, Matt, at 24 years old after having been together since I was seventeen. We already owned a house, and by the way of society the next step for us was children. I got pregnant December of 2004, which ended in a miscarriage very early on in the pregnancy. In January of 2006 we welcomed our first little girl, Madelyn. She came to us after a very long nine months of a challenging pregnancy. My five-foot frame did not carry the 50 pounds I gained very well. I was never one of those cute pregnant girls who are 'all belly'. I carried this child from head to toe, even growing three shoe sizes. At work one day during this pregnancy, I had been hitting up the vending machine for some chocolaty goodness. Realizing I had forgotten my change in the machine, I quickly turned around and went back into the cafeteria only to overhear three women discussing how I was carrying this baby in my ass. I laughed it off as I walked back out the door, and found the nearest garbage can to throw my candy wrapper and my pride into.

The one benefit to all this weight I had tacked on was that I finally saw the big chest I was promised all those years ago coming to fruition! Up to a D-cup, I thoroughly enjoyed my larger boobs, and I wasn't alone. My husband surely wasn't complaining. The confidence I found in my growing breasts was short lived. As I worked hard to lose the baby weight after Maddie was born, I saw my D-cup slowly diminishing to less than what I started with before I got pregnant. Was this a joke? I said to my mom, "You promised me I could have the chest of a real girl after kids." I was sad about 'the girls' shrinking but I, of course, was too preoccupied being Mommy to my baby girl to really care too much.

I had the pleasure of another visit by 'the girls' almost 2 years later when I became pregnant again. Gaining the same 50 pounds back and enjoying my D-cup, this pregnancy mimicked the last one. In 2008, Matt and I welcomed our second little girl, Alexandra. Again, as much as I hoped to keep my large boobs, I watched them disappear over the next year with the baby weight I lost. My dear husband and I love to joke around with one another and my small boobs were always the butt of our jokes. However, my breasts no longer even looked like breasts; they resembled more of a small piece of fruit left too long in the dehydrator.

Little by little I could certainly feel myself becoming more and more self-conscious about my itty-bitty titties. I mean, at least before kids I could say I was a B-cup. Now, I wasn't even sure there was a cup size to describe what was happening underneath my shirt. Why didn't I get to keep my voluptuous breasts after kids like I was promised? I had been duped!

Chapter Two

~ So Many Boobs ~

So here I was, 30 something, a busy working mom of two little girls. Matt had been working as a corrections officer at the county jail for a few years. We both felt tattered and torn by his shift work but we managed. I found myself constantly attempting to find that perfect balance of work and home. It's kind of like playing paddle ball, just when you think you've got things lined up perfectly, the ball veers left and slaps you right in the face. We somehow managed to keep it all together with the help of my amazing mother and some really great friends. It was difficult to say the least; we had lost Matt's mom to a battle with cancer two weeks after Lexie was born. At Lexie's most difficult moments, I like to think that my mother-in-law still resides within her just to get back at Matt for what he may have put her through growing up: a silent revenge of sorts.

Having been with Matt since I was seventeen, a homeowner at 23, married at 24, and two kids by 28, I thought I had life all figured out. For a short while anyway. Amongst all the madness as a mom, one of the things we tend to loose is ourselves, right? By the time Lexie was three I found myself questioning, "Is this all there is to life?" Work, kids, cleaning…. eat, sleep repeat! I wasn't sure I could do that, I needed something more. Something just for me but I just wasn't sure what that something was! By this time, I had decided in order to spend more time with Matt; I'd join the gym. Working out and lifting weights was something he enjoyed doing so I figured I would give it a try. The gym provided daycare so the kids were covered and it was like a date. Matt would ask me to come try weight lifting with him but my response was always the same, "I don't want to look like a guy!" However, while I would be bouncing from elliptical to treadmill watching the clock, I could see Matt in the weight room with the guys. No matter how long we stayed it never seemed like enough time

13

for him, so why was I so bored? At that moment, I promised myself I would attempt to "hit the weights" with Matt.

As we arrived at the gym the next time, we split off into our respective locker rooms to change. When I came out of the locker room, I followed like a little duckling behind my husband to the weight area. He was pleasantly surprised and seemed so excited I was willing to give this a try. Matt was a great teacher, he started me off slowly with light weights and taught me proper form. Luckily, I did have some clue because of my background in Occupational Therapy. I had spent the last several years teaching injured people how to independently use their bodies again. I just never imagined it would feel so good to be challenging myself and my body with these weights. I quickly fell in love. I was in love with the way bench-pressing resembled life. Carefully placing the weight on either side, preparing my body on the bench, bringing that weight down toward my chest and then using all I had to lift that weight back up. Each time I focused on my breath to help me lift heavier and heavier. That bar was like all life's stresses that weighed heavy on my chest and with each exhale and lift I could let go of whatever was on my mind. I was hooked!

My competitive nature was churning inside me, though. Challenging myself to lift the same weight my husband lifted was no longer fulfilling the desire in me. While at the gym one day I said to Matt, "I want to compete in something regarding weight lifting." I'm not sure he knew the severity of how he would pay for what he said next but he replied, "Maybe you should look at figure competitions." I had no idea what that was but Matt said, "Let me take you to a show and let you see what it's all about."

Within a few short weeks I found myself walking arm and arm with Matt into a High School auditorium that smelled of spray tan and sweat. As I looked around all I saw were muscles. Men with big muscles, women with big muscles, women who looked like men with big muscles; muscles everywhere and I was in awe! *What it must take for someone to look like this*, I thought! As I took a seat next to Matt in the auditorium, I was completely intrigued. The lights! The stage! I could feel a burning starting inside of me as the thumping of the music began. As the bright lights shown down on the stage, the figure contestants began to line up. I couldn't take my eyes off of these women. They were muscular but still feminine. Each one had a dark tan that had been strategically sprayed on their perfected bodies. Their hair was done beautifully, and each woman had jewelry and clear heels to finish off their look. Bikinis that glimmered in the hot stage lights, each one more brilliant than the next. As each woman posed to accentuate her muscles all I could envision was myself up on that stage. I didn't belong here in the audience, watching these women. I wanted to be up on that stage, I wanted to do what it took to stand there and show off my hard work.

Turning to Matt I said, "I am going to do a figure competition." He smiled; having already known my competitive nature would drive me to want to be part of this. "There is someone I want you to meet." he said to me. Taking my hand and leading me across the room, he brought me to a petite, gorgeous, blonde, muscular woman. "You must be Angelica." he asked this woman. "Yes, I am, she smiled warmly, her eyes bright and blue. "This is my wife, Tara. We want to know if you would coach her to compete in figure competitions?" Her smile grew and we spoke for a while about how Matt found her and learned of her own successes as a figure competitor, having just earned her pro card in the sport. Angelica had no idea that we would approach her that day but she and I immediately became close and she agreed to coach me on my journey to becoming a figure competitor. When I decided to compete, I didn't really have a clue what this would involve but with my competitive spirit I knew I would do whatever needed to be done.

For the next several months I lifted weights like it was my job. Only, it wasn't my job. I was working almost full time hours and still finding time for 1.5-2 hours a day at the gym. I loved every minute of training. Lifting was therapeutic and Matt spent a lot of time helping to train me. Angelica wasn't local to me so I only had the opportunity to train with her once a month. Most of our time was spent Skyping and mostly with me in my underwear so she could see my progress. I was constantly taking pictures of myself to document the changes in my physique. The transformation was an impressive one. I had a good foundation to build upon thanks to all my years of dancing and the fact that muscle has memory.

Armed with a very clean, strict diet, I was turning into one of those many women I aspired to be on that stage. Months went by and Angelica and I had set a date for my first show. I was filled with excitement as the time approached. By the time we reached this point, I was spending 1.5-2 hours a day doing cardio and about an hour a day lifting weights. I was hyper-focused on my goal, spending much of my day envisioning myself on that stage. I practiced posing nearly every time I passed by a mirror. There was a bikini and heels and pretty jewelry that had been purchased and I had eaten enough fish and asparagus for a lifetime. The week of my first show I was

17

down to my goal weight of about 106 pounds on my five-foot frame. My body fat was on point and all that was left to do was continue with my cardio, eat tilapia like it was the only food left on earth and focus on my goal.

My family was supportive through this entire long and grueling process, listening to me complain about yet another carb cut from my meal plan and standing over the garbage crying over a hot dog or piece of pizza that was tossed away. *God, what I would have given for a slice of pizza*, I thought to myself as I wept over the perfectly good food in the garbage. At my weakest moments during my training, I would silently walk to the garbage and find something salvageable, like a piece of pie or half eaten cookie. I would place the delicious goodness in my mouth and slowly chew, savoring the flavor of these forbidden foods. Just as I was about to swallow, I would spit everything out back into the garbage. "What are you doing." Maddie would say to me. Knowing she hadn't seen me take the food but surely she heard me spitting into the garbage, "I had a funny taste in my mouth and needed to spit it out," I would reply. That always seemed to be enough of an explanation for her innocent 6-year-old mind. I was always relieved too, never wanting to explain why her mother would be dumpster diving right here in our own kitchen. I was hungry and it made me very cranky, so it was no secret to my family that my restrictive meal plan was taking its toll on me. We all saw an end in sight as the big day arrived.

Show day! My first show was in April of 2013 in New York at the Metropolitan. Matt and I drove through Friday night madness into Long Island the night before to stay with Angelica and her husband. Sleep did not happen that night. It was a mix between excitement and the loud, out-of-sync snoring that was happening on opposite sides of the house. As I lay in the dark on the air mattress that night, all I could think of was my posing and what it was going to feel like to be up on that stage showing off all my hard work. By morning my nerves had kicked in and I was less than excited to ingest what would be my last meal of tilapia and asparagus for at least a short while until my next show.

We arrived at the venue and it was packed. The familiar smell of spray tan and sweat got my heart rate pumping. *I made it*, I thought to myself. Pride was oozing out of me and I was elated to be at the show. In my robe, I was taken to a room for the infamous spray tan. This was the secret key to showing off the perfect physique. The spray tan had to be on-point in order for the lights to work their magic. If the tan was just right, the lights would accentuate all the right curves and striations of your muscles. This is why the spray tanning process was taken so seriously in the bodybuilding world. No one wanted to work their ass off for months, only to be up on stage and not be accentuated properly. I was prepared for this process, or so I thought.

Angelica was great and told me exactly how things would happen and also just how to 'landscape' prior to this day so I was ready. I made sure there was no chance to be in my rear pose, showing off my glute/hamstring tie-in and out pops a stray pubic hair. No one wants to be 'that girl.' As the other girls and I waited in line like cattle, we all sized one another up and down. I myself was imagining how lean and muscular each girl was under their silk robe compared to me. Occasionally, we would smile at one another but I followed the lead of the other girls. I'm a social person and wanted to make small talk in this awkward line up but noticed there wasn't much chit-chat amongst the group, so I kept to myself.

Quietly standing as proud as could be in my black silk robe about to embark on my first spray tan, I was elated to experience everything this journey had to offer. As I became next in line, I could feel the excitement building. This was getting real. They called me into the tan room, and I had my own little booth. The first thing I noticed was that the men and women doing the tanning were like busy bees, buzzing around the room, herding us cattle in and out as fast as they could. *Wait, MEN and women doing the tanning?* I thought to myself. I am not sure why I hadn't anticipated the possibility of a man tanning me. In fact, I'm sure Angelica mentioned it to me, but as I entered my own little booth, I turned to face the guy who would be making me fifteen shades darker than my usual pasty-white color.

I stood facing out toward the center of the room. There was no door to close or curtain for that matter, the booth was simply three curtains to block the spray from getting onto the person to the sides and back of you. "Drop your robe," the man said to me. My eyes must have been as big as moons as I looked around the room and thought, *drop my what?* However, knowing he wasn't going to have the time or patience to ask again, I did as I was asked. I dropped my robe to the floor and stood in front of him completely naked. He immediately began to get to work on spraying in what seemed like a very routine order for him. I was careful to not make eye contact as all I could think was, "I don't even have pubic hair!" As he sprayed, my eyes were met by the same eyes I waited in line with. You know, that line I thought was so awkward a minute ago. That line now had nothing on this moment. I was by no means shy and I was no stranger to having to be naked in strange places. As a competitive dancer I was familiar with quick costume changes backstage. However, those times I usually had my mother or dance teacher holding a sheet in front of me as to not be completely exposed. This was the most vulnerable I had ever felt. "Arms up, arms down, spread your legs, bend over," this man had to be sure he got the spray into all my nooks and crannies. I blankly followed his instructions having attempted to mentally remove myself from this situation.

I noticed that in addition to the eyes staring back at me in that room, there were also tons of breasts. I had never seen so many breasts in my life! Bigger breasts, smaller breasts, crooked breasts and most of them fake. All of them beautiful, I thought. I found myself staring at all these tan women with these beautiful boobs. It wasn't in a sexual way but in an envious fashion. Did I need boobs to win? Did I fit in here? Did I work hard enough? Am I as muscular as the next girl? All these doubts seem to flood my head so much so that I hadn't even realized my spray tan man was handing me my robe and attempting to send me on my way. I donned my robe, picked my pride up off the floor, and shook off my feelings of doubt to go meet Angelica and get ready for show time.

The next hour went fast and I was grateful to be free of the uncomplimentary thoughts I was having in the tanning booth. I was busy getting prepped, donning my blue shiny bikini, clear heels and bling jewelry. Angelica had done my hair and makeup and before long I felt absolutely stunning. They called my height class to the backstage area. They quickly briefed us on how things go on stage, and within minutes the music started. There I was, standing with other women who had worked just as hard as I had to get there that day but in my head it was only me.

The bass of the music drowned out the feeling of my racing heart inside my chest. I focused on the words of the song thumping loudly through the speakers around me. One by one, each girl took her turn stepping out to the stage to do individual posing. I was ready. I had practiced my posing every day for months. I was next! I could see the judges from here. Just like Angelica said, they were not looking at the girl on stage, they were staring at *me*. She warned me that they would look at stage right to see who the next competitor was and she was correct. Oh my God, I was sure I was going to puke on stage. I stood just as I was told. Going over the list in my head, right leg in front of left, toe pointed out slightly, chest up, abs tight, flaring my lats. What I wasn't counting on was the shaking. Head to toe I was shaking-with nerves or excitement I wasn't sure. Still focused on the lyrics of the music, "Go," the backstage manager says to me. This was it. This was the moment I had sacrificed so much for. The shaking stopped as I strutted myself to front and center stage under those lights. My eyes met each of the judges one at a time and with every quarter turn I took, I breathed through every pose just as I was taught. I felt at home on this stage, under these lights and it felt amazing.

That year I competed in three figure competitions; back to back shows, all within two months of each other. This meant there was no break from the tilapia and asparagus and my mood reflected the lack of calories I was ingesting. I was, however, beyond committed to my program. Angelica knew I had a goal in mind, and she was an amazing coach to get me to that stage on point every time. My body type, however, was never one of a naturally lean state. It took a lot of cardio as well as counting and weighing every ounce of food I ate to assure I would be ready for the stage. Each show required the same amount of spray tan in the same awkward tanning booth, but by the third show, I didn't really think about standing naked in a room full of people. I was too busy thinking about the rice cake and peanut butter I would reward myself with at the end of the day! Three shows and several trophies later, I was feeling so empowered by the way I was able to sculpt my body. I wanted more of this. I was hooked.

Off-season was one of enjoying more calories and gaining some strength back to lift heavy again and gain some more muscle. Eating and lifting was what I loved, so this wasn't difficult for me. Matt and I had the chance to spend some time lifting together again and my moods were more manageable thanks to the increased caloric intake. By the time prep season came around I had put on a fair amount of muscle and Angelica felt I was ready to get on stage with an even better 'package' this time. My hyper focused behavior slowly began to resemble an obsession, but I never acknowledged that. Looking back now I had pushed most of my friends away because I didn't have time for anyone who didn't live in the gym with me. My girls became used to playing in the basement at night so I could be on my stepper getting the remainder of my cardio in. "Mommy, watch me... Mommy, look at me." Yes, yes I see you, I'd say, fully aware I was not paying attention to them but trying to engage my glutes with each step I took. Kids are resilient though, and thank god for that and the lack of memory at their young age, or they may fully resent me for all the times I wasn't there for them when I was training.

I competed in three more competitions the following year. Same story as the year before, all three shows right in a row. Angelica, Matt and I all agreed: if I was prepping for a show, I should get as much out of the training as possible. At this point there was a boom in the fitness industry, and it seemed that the amount of competitors had tripled from the previous year. Competition was stiff. There were a ton of girls, each one more muscular, lean and beautiful than the next. Even with all the extra supplements and additional cardio time we added into my prep, I was not as confident going into these three shows than the year before. In fact, I felt my confidence melting away slowly over the course of the two months I competed that year. I found myself obsessing over exactly what the judges were looking for. Did I need to grow my lats? Did my quads need more definition? Was my glute/hamstring tie in good enough? Were my shoulder caps rounded enough? Did I need big beautiful boobs like all these other women had? These were the thoughts that clouded my mind both on and off the stage. The confident, elated woman who strutted across the stage the year before had vanished. The woman I had become was no longer confident at all and was questioning everything about herself.

With each show that year I became less and less alive. By the end of the third show, Angelica and I knew I needed a break. I gained a lot of weight back right away after that last show. I was enjoying a lot of the foods I had deprived myself of over the past few months and finally began getting my period again. My hormones felt as if they had been on the crazy train and both they and I were glad things were leveling out. I was still working out, but found myself enjoying it more again since I wasn't so focused on a specific goal. The one thing that stuck with me however was counting my calories.

Although I had no plans to compete again I still worried about the weight I had gained after my show. I found myself continuing to weigh my food and count each almond out into the container. Stepping on a scale became a favorite past time of mine even after I had gotten the extra few pounds off. As I found myself yet again standing over the garbage can, spitting out a cookie after frantically chewing it before the girls could see me, I thought to myself, *I've acquired the eating disorder I escaped all those years ago in my dance days.* I kept these little compulsions to myself justifying them in my head as 'in case I decide to compete again,' I won't have as much prep to do. Deep down though, I knew competing again would throw me over the edge. I just wasn't ready to admit it.

27

Chapter Three

~ My Treasured Chest ~

Three years I gave to bodybuilding. Angelica went on to have a very successful career in online editing for various fitness magazines. She decided to stop both competing herself as well as coaching other girls in the industry. She was supportive of my decision to stop competing, although I always liked to say I would get on that stage again someday. "Maybe when I am old enough to compete in the Masters Division," I would say with a smirk. Matt and I continue to remain close with her and her husband. She was more than my coach; she was a mentor and a friend. You can't spend countless hours skyping half naked while she analyzes every inch of your body and not form a close bond.

It took me quite a while to begin to feel like myself again after my three years of training and competing. The illusion of bodybuilding is real: those bodies look like perfection, but on the inside they are broken down and crying for help. My ego had taken a big hit as well. Although my body was recovering, my mind was still filled with doubts. I was able to find a nice balance of work/home/gym, and my body was happy staying at a consistent pace of eating clean most days but indulging now and again. Visions of breasts haunted me, though. I had worked for a long time to change my body, and I realized the one thing I had no control over changing was the fact I still had the chest of a 10-year-old boy. I didn't fill out a dress, I didn't think I looked feminine in a bikini, and I didn't even really need a bra. I would always envision the moments in those tanning rooms, all those boobs staring at me. *Wouldn't it be fun to fill out a dress*, I would think to myself. "Having something more than saggy skin with a nipple to offer my husband in our most intimate times." Why couldn't I be like those girls?

I remember talking to Matt about the subject. I told him all the ways I felt inadequate as a women due to having such small breasts. "I have changed my whole body through diet and exercise," I said, "but this is the one thing I cannot change, or can I?" Similar to when he knew I would need a coach to get me to that figure stage, Matt got to work on researching the best doctors and the best implants available. He used the power of the Internet and word of mouth to find me a great surgeon and within weeks we had a consultation lined up. I wasn't nervous, I was confident this was a safe decision because I had taken the necessary steps in meeting with two of my doctors prior to this consultation. Both doctors had assured me that implants had become so popular, so perfected, and thousands of women had them. I was assured that they were perfectly safe.

As the plastic surgeon greeted us that day, he found Matt and I in the exam room fondling various types of implants and laughing with one another like silly school kids. There were big implants, small implants, saline ones, and silicone, even implants with a rough outer shell. So many to choose from! This was getting exciting. He was a nice man, my surgeon. I knew this because in the waiting room I sifted through an entire photo album of him helping patients overseas, pro-bono, to repair their facial birth defects. Giving the less fortunate a chance at a better life, for free! *This had to be a good man*, I thought to myself. He thoroughly explained the process of implanting as well as the small risks I could face of losing nipple sensation and experiencing capsular contracture. Capsular contracture as it was explained to me, was the hardening of the scar tissue that forms around the implant. Through the multitude of implants, we learned that capsular contracture chances were lower with a textured implant, the one with the rough outer surface. It was a pricier implant but if it meant my only risk was loss of nipple sensation with these "lifetime devices" then we were willing to pay the extra money.

'Before' pictures were taken, and for privacy reasons they leave your face out of the photo. I figure if someone photo shopped a ten-year-old boy's face onto my body; no one would notice any difference. Then it came time to choose what size implants would be right for me. The benefit to this surgeon was he had a fancy machine that would digitize your photo and measurements, and then with the touch of a few buttons, it would show you what you could look like with implants. *Wow*, I thought as he slowly increased the size on the monitor. "I look like a real girl," I remember saying. We all chuckled as we went back and forth adding and omitting cc's to the implants on the screen. I made it very clear that I didn't want my implants to look like balloons; I wasn't getting them to flaunt them. All I wanted was enough to fill out a shirt. We decided on 370 cc's, which would take my small A to a C cup. The textured implants would not only lessen my chances of capsular contracture but also assure that they would not slip and end up in my armpits. The last decision was that they would be a teardrop shape implant. This was because I didn't want my breasts to be up in my chin. The teardrop implant would guarantee me a natural shape. We signed on the dotted line and set a surgery date.

Before surgery, I spent a lot of time visualizing what I would look like after the surgery. Similar to the girls at the competitions getting tanned, I was going to have perky boobs that would stand at attention no matter what. I had slight anxiety about how to tell my daughters what was happening to Mommy. I didn't feel it was fair to assume they would be oblivious enough not to notice when Mom grew breasts overnight. So I sat them down, Maddie, nine and Lexie, seven. I explained how after I gave birth to them, my boobs got a lot smaller, and I found a doctor who could make them bigger again. It sounded innocent and benign enough that they didn't ask too many questions.

I also experienced a slight guilt before the surgery. I had two dear friends who had battled breast cancer and survived a double mastectomy, expanders, and reconstructive surgery. Experiencing a lot of guilt, I reached out and told them what I was doing and my reasoning behind it. They were very gracious and never judged, but deep in my soul I was feeling that if I was lucky enough not to be the one with breast cancer, I should just leave well enough alone. However, those thoughts were fleeting and after speaking with my friends, I felt I needed to let go of this guilt I was placing on myself.

April 3, 2015 was the scheduled day to receive my breast implants. When the day arrived, I was nervous about having surgery, but equally excited about finally needing a bra. The Valium took the edge off on the way to surgery, and I don't really remember much of that morning. I do remember getting into the OR and seeing my surgeon. As the anesthesiologist was working to get me to sleep, I was busy joking with my surgeon if he remembered both implants. "Yes, I have two implants for you," he said as he grinned at me. The OR nurse above my head was losing her sense of humor waiting for the anesthesia to kick in, and the last thing I remember was her yelling at me to be quiet and go to sleep.

I woke up to the beep of the heart monitor and a loud moaning in the distance. Struggling to open my eyes, I began to feel a lot of pressure on my chest, almost as if someone was sitting there. I looked down, I saw no one. There was no one sitting on my chest and there was no one to tell me where that moaning was coming from. As I finally managed to open my eyes, the moans turned to groans and this poor woman was asking for her husband. Good Lord. *Someone quiet this woman and get her husband*, I thought to myself. Feeling myself beginning to come-to, I realized the moans and groans were coming from me. I felt like I had been hit by a truck and the after effects were two swollen balloons on my chest. I suppose the moaning got annoying enough that someone fetched my husband and he came into my recovery space within a few minutes. The jokester he was, he decided this moment needed to be captured on video so he pretended to interview me. "How do you feel?" he asked as he pointed his cell phone camera in my direction. My response was simple, "My boobs hurt," I said while sipping my ginger ale and taking a small nibble on a graham cracker. "What do you want to tell everyone?" he asked. "Just do it," I replied. "Say goodnight, Momma," Matt told me. "Goodnight, Momma," I mumbled as I painfully put my head back on the pillow.

He shut the camera off and the surgeon walked into the room. "Surgery went well, and you're free to go home now," he exclaimed. This was music to my ears as I was sure I would feel much better on my own couch. Matt assisted me in getting dressed, into my sweat pants, crocs, and zip up sweatshirt. The pulling and stretching in my chest was awful, and I was thankful when the wheelchair arrived and I didn't have to walk all the way down to the lower level of the hospital.

Again, Matt assisted me to step up into my Jeep Wrangler and once I was there, I was out. I don't know if it was the drugs or the pain but I don't remember getting home that day. All I remember was pulling into the driveway being thankful to be home, and also thankful that I didn't puke because I was very nauseous. Matt was so helpful in taking care of me, even sleeping on the couch next to me in case I needed anything at night.

I distinctly remember the second night: I awoke in such a panic. I had been dreaming a wolf was chasing me and I was running and running and I couldn't get away. When I tripped and fell, the wolf was standing on my chest and I couldn't breathe. I was screaming, "Get off me, get off me." My cries were so loud, I woke Matt up out of a deep sleep and he had to calm me down. Although this dream was fictional, the crushing feeling in my chest was not imagined.

At my two day follow up appointment, the surgeon said there would be some pain, but that I would be up and around in a few days. He also unwrapped my compression cover that day and revealed 'the girls' for the first time. Wow, they were absolutely the most perfect breasts I had ever seen! They were not too big and they had a fantastically natural shape to them. Just as I had requested, they were not sitting up in my chin. He assured me the swelling would go down and they would become softer in a few short months. He sent me on my way with my new treasured chest filled in a large size sports bra. Having seen the work of art on my chest, the pain subsided for a short while due to the excitement of thinking about wearing clothes I could have only dreamed about filling out just a few days ago.

While driving home that day, my bra busted open. Bam! Just like that, 'the girls' came out of the open front bra. This was certainly a first for me. "Good Lord!" I shouted as I motioned for Matt to pull over. We had a good laugh on the side of the road that day as Matt put the Jeep in park, came around to my side and helped me squeeze myself back into the bra. I was sure exploring uncharted territory here.

The third day after surgery was Easter. I had mustered up the strength to get in the car with Matt and the girls and drive the 30 minutes to my mom's house. I remember I was there that day, but I don't remember much else. I was in a fog and figured it was due to all the pain I was feeling. The surgeon did mention that after all the bodybuilding I had done, my pec muscles were very tight. I had asked for my implants to be placed under the muscle and therefore he had to do a lot of stretching to get my implants in place. I assumed this much pain was normal for the amount of stretching my skin was doing to accept these new boobs.

It was a while before I was comfortable and the extreme stretching feeling subsided enough for me to be functional again. Although I knew several women who had also just had breast augmentation surgery and were out and about within 3-4 days after surgery, I was trying to be patient with my recovery. Knowing that everyone is different; once I healed I would be able to live a full confident life with my 'safe lifetime devices.' Returning to work just a week after surgery was rough and I was grateful to work with a supportive bunch of women who understood when I had reached my limit and they stepped in to help.

Limits were new to me. This was not something I was used to having, and I was confident it would only be a matter of time until I returned to my life without limitations. I just needed to get past this part; the part where it hurt to lay on my belly, where I was struggling to recover from the anesthesia, and was always short of breath. I was confident that this would be temporary and I would be enjoying my new figure in no time.

"How are you feeling?" the surgeon asked me at my one-month follow up appointment. "I feel OK," I replied. This wasn't a lie, but I had no other real explanation for exactly how I was feeling, so I felt that 'OK' was the most appropriate response. The doc began his usual exam, measurements and palpation of my breasts and axilla area. "Breasts are softening," he dictated to his nurse as she jotted notes into my chart. While I lay back on the exam table with my arms up in the air, all I could think of was my armpits. Thank God I have an amazing husband who was willing to shave them for me. I had been struggling to lift my arm up long enough to shave them thoroughly myself. "I can't go to the doctor with hairy pits," I remember saying to him the night before. So there we were in the bathroom with my arm resting on the top of his head and his face in my armpit, meticulously removing each hair. Maddie walks into the bathroom with a confused look on her face: "Daddy's helping me," I say. "OK," she replied and left without question.

Although I was wrapped in this daydream, I was conscious enough to realize the doctor was palpating a long while up in my armpit, both of them. I could tell he was concentrating on something as he turned to his nurse for dictation and says, "Slight lymphadenopathy on both the left and right sides." My worry about hairy pits seemed childish now as I struggle to take a deep breath. He asks me to sit up, and as I cover myself back up with my pink gown I wait for him to explain what it was he was feeling around for. Impatiently, I ask, "What is lymphadenopathy?" He explained to us that it's just a simple irritation of the lymph nodes and it's perfectly normal after surgery. I know he was hoping I would focus only on the words: simple and normal. However, I have worked in healthcare long enough to hone in on 'irritation and lymph nodes'. I knew that lymph nodes are those small bumps that arise when we are sick and their purpose is to contain immune cells that help your body fight infection. *Was my body infected?* I thought to myself. "Why would they be swollen?" I asked. He rattled off something about my body recognizing my implants as foreign objects and that in some time the lymph nodes would settle down. "I'll see you again in six months, he said, and I will check them then." Sensing my anxiety, he tenderly touched my hand and said, "Please don't worry." I silently gathered up my things, got my shirt on, and Matt and I left the office after making my next appointment.

In the car Matt attempted to keep me calm. Knowing me so well, he held my hand and assured me that the doctor said this was normal and not to worry. *Worry*, I thought, *I'm not worried. I'm terrified!* People's lymph nodes swell when they get sick or when they have cancer, and I am not sick. So what does this all mean? Why 'Foreign objects?' Those two words kept ringing in my head. All the way home, over and over again, all I could think of were the words, "foreign objects." Up until now, all the doctors I consulted with about getting breast implants always referred to them as 'perfectly safe lifetime devices'. Never once had anyone called them 'foreign objects,' and yet that made perfect sense to me now that it was being said out loud. I was just disappointed in myself for not seeing them in that light before today, after these 'foreign objects' have already been implanted in me.

That night as I sat at home, I had a talk with my body. I told it how we had already survived two C-sections, an umbilical hernia surgery, and that we just needed time to heal from this surgery. I decided the best thing for me was to continue to focus on healing completely from surgery and not to worry about anything. I began to relax, let the worry go, and enjoy my new body. At least that's how I made it look on the outside.

Chapter Four

~ Well These Are FUN!

... Or Are They? ~

2015

The first several months after getting my implants were an adjustment period. I began to live through all the things I had heard about but never experienced. Like boob sweat. I am not a sweaty person by any means. In fact, I think I suffer from some weird aliment where I don't sweat enough; especially on my face, which is why I have always struggled with some acne. This though, was like nothing I have ever experienced. About 30 seconds into my workout, the sweat would be pouring out from between 'the girls'. I have no shame; I would be that girl jamming my towel in between my boobs to soak it up and whine about how annoying it is. I hadn't yet become totally comfortable with my breasts. For instance, I didn't realize that when you have implants your headlights are always on... and I mean *always*. I suppose some girls enjoy showing them off, but that wasn't me. I spent many bathroom trips at the gym attempting to fold up toilet paper and put it in my bra to block my nipples. It never worked: I always ended up looking like I had some weird square areola. Bathing suits were exciting to fill out even though it took me a while to find some that didn't expose too much.

Looking back now, I realize I was attempting to make fake look completely real, which was an impossible task. I did however truly enjoy filling out a tee shirt. Any kind of tee shirt made me feel happy. There is something about having a fuller chest that creates an illusion of also having a smaller waist, and who doesn't love some good curves?

That spring and summer of 2015, we attended three weddings. I enjoyed shopping for new dresses and even utilizing old ones in my closet, basking in the fact I filled them out better now. It was fun to feel like a "real girl". On the dance floor, I felt some newfound confidence that wasn't there before. I used to always find myself looking at the other women in the room, envious of the fact they filled out their dress like a woman. Now here I was, bustin' it up on the dance floor and I was that woman. I filled out my dress, and it felt good! My six-month appointment was approaching, and if I told you I wasn't obsessively digging in my armpit to check my lymph nodes, I would be lying to you. I was checking them, daily.

Assuming my position on the exam table at my next appointment in my pink gown, the doctor walks in to greet me. "How are you doing?" he asked. *How was I doing? Do I tell him I obsessively check my lymph nodes? Do I mention that I am still peeing all the time since having anesthesia? Do I tell him the elephant he placed on my chest is still sitting there since April?* "I feel good," I say. As he began to start his exam he looks at me and says, "Your face is very broken out." He was right. Three days after surgery, I had an acne flare up. Being that I had a tough time coming out of anesthesia, I assumed the acne was due to that. As he performed his exam, he asked how I liked my new boobs. I told him how happy I was to be filling out my clothes and dresses, and that he did a good job giving me exactly what I had asked for. His hands began to manipulate around my axilla and again he hovered over these two spots for a longer time. He turned to the nurse and said, "Slight adenopathy on both sides." I sat up and as I held the tears back, thinking they would have relaxed by now, I asked, "Why are they still swollen?" He gave the same blanket statement about my body recognizing them as foreign objects and needing time to adjust. "I'm worried," I mumbled. Although he again attempted to assure me that this was normal, I felt equally as uneasy about it as I did the first time. "Everything looks good," he said again. "Come see me in six months and I'll check your lymph nodes again. However, if you experience any swelling on either side, please come in right away."

My heart sunk. Why? Why were my 'perfectly safe lifetime devices' causing me such anxiety? Again, I silently gathered up my things, got my shirt on, and I left the office after making another six-month appointment. This time, I cried all the way home.

Life taught me at, an early age, that when times get tough, you put on your bravest face and keep forging on. So that's just what I did. Although I had a sinking feeling in my gut every time I checked my lymph nodes, I managed to suppress my anxiety most days. Occasionally, I would say to my mother or to Matt, "I'm worried this isn't normal." However, similar to how I was trained to wear my brave face, I was also trained to trust doctors. They were the experts. The men and women who would diagnose and treat whatever aliments may arise. The doctors have the answers, so of course if the plastic surgeon was telling me this was normal, I was worrying for nothing. I decided to let go. I had beautiful new breasts that I deserved to enjoy and I was determined to do so.

2016

I began a new job that second year, working full time. Previously, I was commuting further but working 24 hours per week. Increasing to 40 hours was a lot for me to adjust to and I felt it. Slowly, I found myself being too tired from the extended hours to have energy for the gym. I would drive past on my way home and attempt to pep talk myself into the parking lot. Most days though, I drove right past the gym and headed home. At this point in Matt's career we were thrilled to have him on the day shift, so I didn't have to handle the girls alone at night. I liked my new job a lot; I've always enjoyed working with the developmentally disabled population. The clients bring me a lot of joy, and so does helping them. It was a large facility though, and that meant a lot of employees.

My memory continued to fail me so I carried a notebook to jot down the names of people I met. Later, I would study them at the end of the day. I would feel so proud after learning several new names. Within a few months, I had learned so many names and made lot of new friends. My new friends didn't even have a clue that I had breast implants. The size I chose was big enough to fill out my clothes but not big enough that they looked un-natural. I had chosen to tell about three people over the course of the first year I worked there.

The first half of my first year at my job, I had missed some days at work for the normal things you expect; sick kids, snow days, a common cold. The second half of the year, I had some things I needed to take care of for myself, things I had been ignoring for a while. Ever since my surgery, I noticed I was still peeing all the time, about every 45 minutes to an hour. It was such a nuisance both at work and when I was out with my family. I saw an endocrinologist for this, thinking that I was possibly diabetic. I could only assume this would have been caused by my crazy dieting while I was training for my bodybuilding. My bloodwork came back normal on all counts and he assured me I was not diabetic. This was a relief to me, however, it didn't answer the question 'why' and the frequent urination continued. Even my gynecologist agreed that after a woman has children it is normal to pee more frequently. I would also ask her at my annual exam each year to check my lymph nodes as they were forever in the back of my mind. She would palpate them after doing my breast exam, and tell me they were small. If the surgeon wasn't concerned, she assured me I was fine. "My period seems to be changing," I would say at my exam. "You could be in the beginning stages of menopause," she would reply. Each year I would think to myself, beginning menopause at 36, 37 years old? If she said it was possible, then I guess I would just have to suck it up and deal with having my period every three weeks. I succumbed to the fact I was getting older, and this was my new normal. "What about my acne doc," I would ask her. She would assure me that many women suffer from adult acne. "You'll have to see a dermatologist," she would say, as we would end our appointment. So, I did see a dermatologist. Three of them in fact. I tried every oral antibiotic and topical cream/gel/lotion that has ever existed. These things would work for a while but as soon as the dose stopped, I would be back to the large, painful, cyst-type bumps on my face.

By the second half of the second year, I still hadn't really adjusted to my 40 hour a week commitment. I was exhausted all the time. I would live for the weekends, and find myself attempting to muster up the energy to keep up with my family those days. Attempting to keep in touch with old friends from former jobs, I found that I didn't even have the motivation for dinner and drinks. On the days/nights when I did muster up the energy to go out, I found myself making excuses to go home early. I was tired to my core and also felt angst inside me I had never felt before. Most days when I found myself too tired to function at night, I would verbally abuse myself about how I ruined my body with all the training I did a few years prior and how it must have taken a toll on my adrenal glands, thyroid, and hormones. I was beginning to struggle with daily life. I secluded myself from social media because I could no longer tolerate watching all the people I used to work out with continue to have energy when I didn't.

By the end of the second year, it was a successful week at work if I accomplished working my full schedule. Most weeks my absence was due to doctors' appointments or not feeling well. Often times I found myself laughing alongside my co-workers about how I acted like I was 80 years old. Inside, I wasn't really laughing.

2017

My third year with my cohesive silicone gel textured teardrop implants began in April of 2017. "I'm doing OK" or "I'm hanging in there" were my blanket responses for when people asked me how I am doing. I wasn't going to lie: I didn't feel good, ever. To my knowledge, people couldn't tell how sick I was feeling on the inside. I looked healthy with the exception of my acne and my eyes. At this point I was suffering so badly with cystic acne that my face was red and swollen. Most nights, I would have to apply ice to calm the burning while I sat my exhausted ass on the couch. My eyes were telling a story that even I didn't know was churning inside me. They were tired eyes, little slits that felt as though I had weights attached to my thinning eyelashes. Eyes that were so heavy and if you looked close enough you could see that the color of my eyes were different. The blue was less vibrant and the whites were almost a grey color. I often wondered if anyone could tell.

In May of 2017, I made an appointment with my plastic surgeon to discuss a pain in my breast that I began having. "I have been doing this for years, Tara. You have got to trust me when I say you are fine," he said to me. "I am just worried something isn't right," I replied. Assuming I knew what he was talking about, the doctor says to me, "I am guessing you read the article in the newspaper about the rare cancer caused by breast implants?" Suddenly, I felt sick. I definitely couldn't breathe. Did he just say cancer??? A risk of cancer caused by my 'safe lifetime devices'? "No, doc," I stated. I hadn't heard anything about what he was talking about. "OK, well there is a woman who has been diagnosed with a rare form of lymphoma. She believes it's due to her breast implants." He named the cancer with some letters I didn't retain and informed me about how the article ran a few months ago in the newspaper. "There is nothing for you to worry about, Tara," he continued. This rare cancer is linked to textured implants and yours are smooth," he attempted to assure me. Holding back tears, I gently reminded him, "No, my implants are textured." Thinking back at that very moment to the consultations I had with not only this man before me, but also other trusted doctors. "Can breast implants cause cancer or damage my health in any way?" I asked several doctors prior to making my decision to get implants. Having been told by each one that so many women these days get implants and that they are perfectly safe, I was feeling sick to my stomach. I felt lied to and mislead by so many. If I had been aware of even a 1% chance of implants causing me harm, I would have never chosen to get them.

My plastic surgeon made his best attempt at easing my mind with words like "very rare", "don't worry", "one in thousands of women," but I was in a fog. He gave me the link to the article so I could read it for myself, and he said the only reason for me to worry would be if I had swelling in one of my breasts. It was definitely nausea I was experiencing. This was news I wasn't prepared for and after reading the article many times over, I talked myself down by repeating those same key words to myself. *Rare, don't worry, one in thousands of women.* I have since learned that BIA-ALCL stands for Breast Implant Associated-Anaplastic Large Cell Lymphoma. It's a man-made cancer caused by breast implants. It is not a breast cancer, but a cancer caused by your body's immune response to the texture of the implants. After that appointment, I tried to remain calm. I forced myself to stop reading the article. I focused on the fact that it was 'rare', and I hadn't had any swelling like my surgeon spoke of. However, looking for any signs of swelling was added to my daily ritual of obsessively checking my lymph nodes. Wow, these breasts sure were fun?!?

By the middle of my third year with my implants, I was no longer enjoying them at all. Don't get me wrong, they looked amazing, but I was feeling too sick to enjoy anything those days. The gym was a thing of the past; I had no energy to workout nor did I have any strength left to lift weights. It took all I had to carry groceries from the car to the house so weight training was out of the question. When I did muster up the strength to get myself to the gym, I would find myself on the elliptical, daydreaming. Thinking about how tired I was and looking for any excuse to go home and sit on the couch, I would desperately search for a shred of motivation to come light a fire under my ass. With my anxiety at an all-time high, I even attempted to workout at home. Thinking that maybe I was too afraid to be seen in public with my cystic acne, I would force myself to the basement on my stepper. Most days this was unsuccessful as well. I had resigned to the fact my membership dues would just be a yearly donation to the gym.

My sex drive was nonexistent. Prior to my implants I remember thinking how great it would be to not feel self-conscious during intimate times with my husband. I had worked so hard to sculpt my body to look good but my small breasts were out of my control. So here I was waiting anxiously for the amazing changes in libido I was promised; they never showed. It was devastating to me to have spent so much money on these beautiful breasts and not have any drive to utilize them. I couldn't tell Matt how disappointed I was because we were still paying for these 'safe lifetime devices'. After all, I was the one who was sure these boobs were going to bring me happiness and confidence. I couldn't be the one to say I wasn't happy on the inside, which would bring disappointment to more than just me. I just continued to go through the motions.

I wasn't sure if it was the acne or the anxiety, but depression settled in that year. My gynecologist suggested it was my age and being peri-menopausal that had me down and out! I assumed she was right. This must be what it feels like to be 37? Tired, depressed, anxious, in pain, dead on the inside... wow, my perky boobs and I sure were the life of the party!

At each follow up appointment with my plastic surgeon he followed the standard routine of checking my lymph nodes and finding the same result each time. He added the discussion about the BIA-ALCL, and continually told me how rare this was, assuring me that I was safe because I had no signs of swelling. The only addition to that worry was the pain I was continuing to experience. The pain was exclusive to my left side and radiated from my armpit to my nipple. This same pain had brought me to his office just a few short months earlier,

54

but those worries were squashed by the news of possible cancer associated with my implants. "Completely normal," he would assure me. I would be told that I had done too much and that nerve pain was a side effect of my 'perfectly safe lifetime devices.' Less than assured, I would gather my belongings and make my next appointment.

The only difference with this particular appointment in that third year was that I didn't drive home in tears. I found myself in deep thought during my ride home that day. All I could think was 'how could I have done too much'? I don't ever do 'too much' these days; in fact, I don't do much of anything. Feeling like I was barely existing was the level I was functioning at. So how the hell could I have done too much? Why did I feel tired and foggy all the time? Where was all this anxiety I was experiencing coming from? Something was wrong with me? But what?

Chapter Five

~ The Gift ~

We all have those times in our lives that break us, challenge us and change us. It's all according to how you choose to respond to these situations that dictate if you become changed for better or worse. This is your character: it makes you who you are. These moments in time come to us usually when we least expect them. I believe life throws these curve balls for a reason. If you saw them coming, you'd duck, you'd change your position, prepare yourself. The universe waits for you to be unprepared and catch you off guard. This ensures you will be at your most vulnerable and that you'll have the rawest experience possible. You must be broken. Fallen to pieces in order to learn to pick yourself up and figure out how to put yourself together again. And when you do pick yourself up and ask that all too familiar question of "Why Me?" Your answer is in the outcome. The outcome is your reward; the reward is who you become after the storm is over. Being broken is a gift from God, a package you get to slowly unwrap. What you find inside is all up to you. That is the beauty of the gift.

So what happened to me in those days prior to ending up on the bathtub floor, soaked in my own tears? How did I become so broken? It was loss. In that moment I realized I had lost everything I knew. Spending the past three years waiting to love my new body when all it was, was broken. Beaten by whatever was burning inside it that had yet to unveil itself to me. I had lost the ability to mother my children the way they needed me to. The fatigue had plagued me, and I couldn't keep up with my family's needs any longer. A tired wife whose husband needed her with his ever changing work schedule, and I was vacant. I felt dead on the inside. I was a shell of a human being, and the scariest part was I had no idea what was happening to me.

In November of 2017, just three short years after my breast augmentation surgery I found myself and my faith being tested. I had a 'chosen' family member who I was medically responsible for, and he had fallen ill. This was a man who I had met in 2004 at work. A gentle 76-year-old soul with cerebral palsy who was confined to a wheelchair for the 13 years I had known him. As an Occupational Therapist, we teach people how to be as independent as their abilities allow. Little did I know that when I met Chuck, he would teach me more than I could have ever taught him. Although his spastic body didn't always cooperate for him, his mind was sharp and his heart was larger than anyone else I'd ever known. We were family; he adopted me, Matt and the girls as his own and we adored him just the same. He entrusted me with his medical decisions a few years before and on Thanksgiving Day of 2017 he landed in the hospital. I went to him and for days I was with him alongside his sister and niece making decisions that would affect the outcome of his life. If you have ever been chosen by someone to make these decisions for them, it's a responsibility like no other. I tried to be true to his wishes, which we had discussed in length in many heart to hearts we'd had over the years. It's when the decisions are not so black and white that it knocks the wind out of you.

We all did what we knew to be right by Chuck in those weeks and ultimately it was inevitable that we would lose him. The time I spent with him in those days was priceless. Although I had been feeling ill myself, I went to be with him as much as I could. My only regret was that I had let the fatigue get to me so badly, I hadn't had the time I would have liked with him in the past three years. He understood though, and never complained. That was Chuck, always finding the good and never once asking concessions. In those last days, we sat and talked just like we always had. His weakness was making his speech even more difficult to understand than usual, but with mutual patience, I heard him. As we sat by the Christmas tree his family arranged for him, we marveled at the glorious lights and the "Grandpa" ornament Lexie had given him just days earlier when Matt and the girls came to see him. Each day I saw Chuck he would say to me, "What do you want for your birthday?" It was December at this point and he never forgot that my birthday was the 14th. My answer was the same this year as it has been for all the years prior, "Just you." I would say, "Having you in my family's life is all I need." He would smile and giggle and usually give me a thoughtful bracelet or necklace, all of which I cherished.

This was our routine for several days in December and in my heart I didn't want this to end. When I received a call from his doctor on my way to work one morning, I knew it would all be ending soon, even prior to answering the phone. "Come now," she said. On the drive there, I called his family who needed to come from out of state. I needed to keep my mind occupied on something, anything else. He was alert when I arrived, and I was never so grateful to see his big blue eyes smiling at me. His hands were warm under the oversized blue blanket that seemed to make his eyes shine even brighter. "What's new", I said as always when I sat down next to his bed. He smiled and looked up at me with his usual reply; "New York, New Jersey, New England," and we both belly laughed. I was enthralled with the fact he could joke at a time like this. *At a time like this*, I thought to myself. *Maybe he was unaware of what was even happening to him*, I thought. This was a talk I needed to have with him. When he decided he trusted me enough to help make decisions regarding his health when he no longer could, this meant he also trusted me enough to be honest with him about what was happening.

I placed my cool hand on his warm head, standing up so my eyes met his. The only sound in the room was that of a harp playing gentle Christmas notes. "I love you, Chuck," I said. "I don't know why God sent me here all those years ago, but I am so glad he did because you are my family." "Matt, the girls and I love you so much." He smiled, listening intently. "I want you to know that it's time. It's time for you to go be with your Mom and your Dad," I said. Remembering the doctor told me it's good to give a loved one permission, I continued, "It's OK to go, Chuck. Your work here is done and you are amazing." He was quiet for a long time, while I gathered up tissues and collected myself. His eyes, clear as the sky on a spring day, looked up at me. "You were sent here because you are so special to me," he said. Thankful that these words came out so clear, I kissed his forehead. A peace came over me as I saw Chuck's eyes begin to fade. "One more thing," I said to him as I held his hand. "I finally know what I want for my birthday, Chuck," I said gently. His eyes met mine, "I want you to let go and be with God," I whispered.

He said nothing but I knew he had heard me. A short while later he slept. It was the most peaceful sleep I had ever seen. His breaths were shallow, but I found myself mesmerized by the rhythm of them. He didn't wake when I left that night and by morning, he was gone. It was my birthday.

In the days following Chuck's passing, I was numb. Heartbroken for my loss, I began to reflect. The moment I found myself balled up on the floor of my tub, I reflected on all that had happened. In those moments sitting with Chuck while he slowly drifted deeper and deeper into the sheets covering his hospital bed, I remember thinking, 'I am dying, too.' This slow progression of his becoming weaker and weaker was an oddly familiar feeling to me. I had been in denial about how sick I had actually become over the past months. The burning and itching on my face was not normal and no dermatologist had been able to provide any answers to me. I had panic attacks on a regular basis that would wake me from a sound sleep. Sitting alone in the kitchen at 2am debating whether to call my husband at work or 911, I eventually learned how to talk myself down from the anxiety. The constant heart palpations, difficulty catching my breath, the constant pain in my throat, the endless gut issues, the never ending ringing in my ears, there were tons of issues I was having that I had been ignoring for a long time now. Losing Chuck was the push I needed to figure out what was wrong, I was armed with my own special angel watching over and I was dedicated to figuring out what was wrong with me, or die trying.

This was the storm in my life that broke me. I was more broken than ever before and I knew in that moment on the shower floor, I had a choice. I could figure out a way to end my misery, or I could accept that I was being called to walk down a dark, difficult path and accept the challenge. In the moment that I physically picked myself off that floor and dried myself off, I committed to accepting this challenge. I was going to take my life back from whatever was happening inside me because this storm had broken me. God speaks to us and through us in these broken times. His presence filled me that night as I picked myself up off that shower floor, collected myself and walked down the stairs to meet my family. I wasn't alone in the bathroom that night for if I had been, I surely wouldn't have made it out alive.

Chapter Six

~ The Ember Inside Me ~

Matt and I have grown up together these past 21 years, and although I pretended to have myself all together; he saw right through the façade. The night of my broken moment in the shower, he held me. Long after the movie ended and the girls were tucked in bed he held me as I sobbed. "What's wrong, Tara," he asked as I convulsed in his arms. It took a long while for me to catch my breath enough to get any words out. Finally, I responded, "I'm dying, Matt," I replied. Bringing my body out to his arm's length so he could see my face, he locked eyes with me. "You are not dying," he said. I appreciated his attempts at reassuring me, however, in my gut I knew there was something slowly taking the life in me away. I collected myself a bit and wiped my eyes and explained to him how watching Chuck die was a turning point for me. Seeing the weakness take over him made me come to terms with the fact that I had become a shell of who I once was. I didn't even recognize myself in the mirror anymore. The outgoing, fun-loving, energetic wife and mother I once was had slowly died. The women who once craved being center of attention on a stage had disappeared. Now, I was a shy, timid woman who was barely clinging on to her existence and I had to figure out what was wrong with me. "I don't think you are dying, Tara, but I support whatever you feel you need to do," he said to me. Then we slept.

That night I dreamed. Something I hadn't done in a very long time. It was a vivid dream; the kind of dream that feels so real you are physically exhausted in the morning. I was digging. Literally, I was digging through the entire dream. I had a metal shovel with a tattered wooden handle. I was alone. I dug in the dirt for what seemed like hours in my dream that night. I woke up being confused by the dream. *What in the world did that dream mean?* I thought to myself. Although the dream was confusing, I was thankful to have slept through the night for the first time in a while. I had recently begun getting woken up from sleep either by pain in my left breast or joint pain in my hips.

My most recent trip to the dermatologist landed me in a 3-day skin allergy test where she applied 80 patches to my back with various products that could be causing my acne issue. After the test was complete I was informed I was severely allergic to *Thimerosal*, a mercury based product. It wasn't an allergy I was born with, she informed me. This was an acquired allergy, and I was given a list of 'safe' products, and told to stay away from anything with a mercury base. The flu shot and other immunizations could contain Thimerosal, I was told. This was funny to me because I was never one that liked getting the flu shot; I always felt it made me sick. But if I didn't get the flu shot and hadn't had any immunizations in a long time, how was I overexposed to mercury? These were the questions that plagued my mind at 2 am after being woken up by pain. While Matt worked the midnight shift I would wake up alone in the bed and Google medical symptoms in hopes I could find some answers to why my 38-year-old body was failing me. 'Mercury causing acne,' I would Google. Dr Google didn't always have answers for me, and when it did, it played heavily into my anxiety.

"Stop googling," the cardiologist told me. "Your echocardiogram and stress test came back perfectly normal," he assured me. Then why am I out of breath all the time, feel like I can't catch my breath, and hear my heartbeat while I am sleeping? "It's anxiety," he replied. Leaving the office, I was given the names of breathing techniques and yoga to try to decrease my anxiety with a strict order to 'stop googling'. I added the list of techniques to my growing folder of medical files.

More dreams came in the following nights. Only these nights I was not digging. These nights I was swimming or running or biking. Never knowing where I was going and never actually arriving anywhere in my dreams, I was equally confused and exhausted by these dreams. It seemed they were coming to me almost every night. Each night I would be doing an exhausting task in a frantic manner and never knowing where I was going and never actually arriving anywhere. I was being spoken to through these nightly visions but what was the message?

The holidays were upon us and all I wanted was to stay home and be by myself. I was depressed and frustrated that I felt like an old lady and had no answers from any doctor as to why. At this point I would joke with my 'very serious' primary care doctor that I should reserve a standing weekly appointment with him. It was one complaint after another for me. I had prided myself on being a strong, healthy woman in the past so this was very uncharacteristic. "What brings you here today, Mrs. Hopko," he would always say to me when he entered the room. The list of ailments was long during those weekly appointments:

- My throat feels funny, almost like it's swollen on the sides.
- My acid reflux is so bad I don't want to eat anymore.
- I have a constant pain in my throat.
- The pain in my left breast is waking me up at night.
- I've had an enlarged lymph node under my chin for months.

The list kept growing and he would document all my complaints in his trusty laptop. "Doc Alex thinks I'm crazy," I would say to Matt when I would return home. "He doesn't even crack a smile when I joke with him," I would say. Matt wasn't convinced the doctor thought I was crazy. He had known him for years and seemed to have a better read on him than I did. "Doc Alex is just a smart, serious guy but he knows his stuff," Matt always assured me. So I continued to see Doc Alex, all the while, wishing he would crack a smile at my feeble attempts at a bad joke during our visits. I thought back to one appointment where he told me I was due for a tetanus shot and I said, no thank you. "What do you mean, no thank you," he asked, almost puzzled by my response. "I don't like to put anything un-natural into my body if I don't need to," I said. I remember thinking out loud in that very moment and continuing with, "That sounds funny coming from someone with silicone bags in her chest, doesn't it?" He didn't look up from his computer as he documented, 'Patient refused tetanus shot'. I laughed at myself out loud but I distinctly remember those thoughts remaining in my head for a long time after that appointment. I sure did feel like an oxy-moron after I had said it out loud. Here I was attempting to eat clean, live clean and take good care of myself, but almost three years prior, I had chosen to insert silicone sacks into my body, right above all my major organs. Oddly enough it was some of those same organs that were giving me trouble at this holiday season. The rapid heart rate, constant palpitations, difficulty catching my breath; these were the reasons I wanted to seclude myself from everyone, every holiday function. I remember thinking this would be my last holiday here anyway. Convinced that the burning inside me that I couldn't rid myself of was going to take my life before the next Christmas rolled around, I just had to make it through this year.

Unknowing of just how deep that ember inside me had gotten, my supportive family humored me and our only plan for Christmas day was to have my mom come over and hang with Matt, the girls and I. Christmas morning came and when I woke up, I couldn't walk. There was an excruciating pain in my left hip. It hurt to bear weight, to sit, and even to lie down. I managed to survive the girls opening Santa's treasures left under the tree, however, by the time my mom arrived I looked at Matt and begged him to take me to the hospital.

I prayed the entire way that everyone else in the area was having a beautiful Christmas morning, and there would be no wait for me to see the doctor and find out what was wrong. God answered my prayers because we arrived and were taken in immediately. An x-ray was taken. Inconclusive. That was the answer I left the hospital with on Christmas morning. That, and a shot for pain directly into my hip. Along with a prescription for an anti-inflammatory medicine that I couldn't fill because it was a holiday. "Follow up with an orthopedic doctor," the ER doc told me when we left.

I couldn't return to work, I couldn't walk. In fact, I hadn't even slept because the pain was so bad. I followed up with the orthopedic doc and an MRI as requested. By the time I got my MRI results, the shot for pain and anti-inflammatory meds began to work and I began to feel some relief. "Are you sure you didn't fall or have an accident," the orthopedic doctor asked. "I am positive I woke up this way on Christmas morning," I responded. He told me I had tendons that were torn inside my left hip as well as in my lower back. His confusion was just as great as mine. He explained that he could only assume these were old tears from all my years of dancing, but the acute pain didn't make sense if there was no recent injury. If the anti-inflammatory meds worked, I didn't need to follow up with him he told me. However, if they didn't provide the necessary relief, I was to come back and discuss, 'other options'. Within one week after Christmas, I had complete relief and was able to walk, sleep and sit with no trouble. Oddly enough, in addition to the relief I experienced with my hip, I also experience relief from my acne with the anti-inflammatory medication. This sparked my interest and now that Christmas was over, it was time to buckle down and figure out what the hell was happening to me.

The correlation between the anti-inflammatory meds and the clearing of my acne had me thinking there could be an autoimmune issue happening within me. I wasn't getting any answers from the doctors I was being referred to, so against medical advice I turned to Google again. I had a nagging feeling for a short time now that I hadn't shared with anyone else yet; I wasn't ready to hear myself say it out loud. Too many doctors had told me that I was a crazy, hypochondriac, anxious, busy mother and wife who spent too much time on the Internet. I was too afraid of what people would think if they knew my suspicion.

"What happened on Christmas Day?" Doc Alex asked me with some concern in his voice. He is a mild mannered man who has never shown much emotion during our appointments, but the urgency in his voice this day had me concerned. "Spontaneous tears in your tendons are not normal, Tara," he stated. I knew this was a true statement even before he made it. After all, just moments earlier I was inconsolable in the car with my mom, scared this was bone cancer of some sort. As she drove with me to Doc Alex that morning, I cried "Mom, I just feel that the burning inside me is growing and I am so scared because no one can tell me what's wrong." She cried with me that day, she was scared, too, and I knew it, but it felt good to tell her just how scared I was. To acknowledge the ember that was smoldering deep within me made me somehow feel I was one step closer to the answers I needed.

The doctor continued as my foggy brain attempted to focus on his words and recommendations, rather than the urgency in his tone. "Follow up with a rheumatologist," he said. "I want you tested for auto-immune disease because this type of severe joint pain doesn't just happen, there is something else going on," he stated. Not surprised I would be on my way to yet another doctor, I took my referral and my tired, foggy, brain and we left.

A few days before my rheumatologist appointment, the family and I were home keeping warm. Everyone was busy around the house as I sat silently Googling by myself. I needed answers to questions that were churning in my mind. Why the mercury allergy? Why did my acne respond to anti-inflammatory meds? I knew doctors had no answers and I was on my own to figure this out. The Internet is a funny place, and by funny I mean it is designed in such a way that you're blocked from seeing certain information a lot of the time. It is full of so much information but you have got to know what you are looking for. I spent most of my free time researching my symptoms but never found the answers because I wasn't asking the Internet the correct questions. Having pondered how I could have been overexposed to mercury, I had checked all my beauty products with nothing checking out positive. I asked

Google, "What are my breast implants made of?" "What are the side effects of breast implants?" Nothing. The answers were not there, you see, I was asking the wrong questions.

After many, many wrong questions, I finally asked the right one. "Can my breast implants make me sick," I wrote. BINGO! I stumbled upon a website that would have knocked me off my feet had I been standing. It was information that made me feel both nauseous and excited at the same time. This website 'Healing Breast Implant Illness' had the answers to all my questions and confirmed that my suspicions were not crazy. My breast implants were making me ill and I WASN'T CRAZY. A website that was created by a women named Nicole, who had been affected by her implants the same way I apparently was being affected by mine. She gave a huge list of symptoms; to which I could relate to 90% of them. Everything from fatigue, to hair loss and weight gain, to heart palpitations and vertigo, to swollen lymph nodes and acne, to anxiety and depression, pain, food sensitivities, and a large list of other aliments I was suffering from. This information brought me to tears. I couldn't believe my eyes. Not only was I not crazy; I was not alone!

There was no greater feeling than knowing all your efforts were not in vain. Here it was in black and white, Breast

74

Implant Illness (BII). Why had I never seen these words before? Why had none of my doctors ever told me this was a possibility? I consulted with several doctors before getting my 'safe lifetime devices'. I began to grow angry very quickly. I felt lied to. I needed time to process this information and work through the denial I felt creeping up on me.

Funny that once you know just what to ask of the Internet, you get all the information you need. Now that I was armed with the knowledge of Breast Implant Illness, I found numerous websites and YouTube videos with women suffering just as I was. I decided to join several Facebook support groups full of countless women who had been sick to the point of feeling as though they were dying, just as I was. I truly wasn't alone and it was both comforting and sickening all at the same time. All of us women from all around the world had been lied to. I learned that these 'safe lifetime devices' were not safe at all. They are made of 40 different chemicals just on the outer shell alone. These implants are then placed over our vital organs, affecting every important system in our body. *What do I do with this info?* I wondered. I had to tell Matt. I just didn't know how.

I find that it's always easier to have difficult discussions with people when you are in the car. I believe this is because it eliminates the need for eye contact. Telling someone something difficult is always easier when you don't have to look them in the eye, or maybe when you don't have to see the look of disappointment on their face looking back at you. "Can I tell you something without you thinking I am crazy?" I said to Matt while we were in the car together one day. "Sure," he replied nonchalantly. Like ripping off a Band-Aid, I just threw it out there. "I think all my issues are being caused by my breast implants", I said lightly. Without waiting for a response, I continued. "Looking back now, I haven't felt right for the past few years and it all seems to have begun when I had my implants put in." He was quiet for a moment. "I am not going to call you crazy but I am not sure if that is the cause of all this," he said gently. I spent time telling him about the website I had found with all the information Nicole had shared about the toxins released from breast implants, and the autoimmune issues that arise. He listened intently as I told him about the Facebook support group that was started by Nicole, and that there were almost 40,000 members in the group. Each woman had her own story of pain, inflammation, autoimmune diagnoses, hair loss, thyroid, and hormonal issues. The list went on. I shared with Matt just how comforting it felt to hear these other women speak of how they, too, felt as though they were dying. Knowing I was not alone was the only comfort I had. "I believe you, Tara. I know you are not crazy and what you feel is real, let's just see what the rheumatologist says and go from there," Matt said.

"Have you ever heard of Breast Implant Illness," I asked the tall, slender rheumatologist who entered the exam room while I assumed my all too familiar position on the exam table. "No, I have not," he replied. "Well, I think my breast implants are causing an autoimmune reaction in my body and that's why I am here today." Giving me the typical response of, 'Many women have implants for years and I have never heard of anyone complain they are making them ill.' I thought to myself, *just maybe there are thousands more women who ARE ill from their implants; they just don't know what's causing their illness yet.* Unfortunately, these women are led by doctors to just treat the symptoms and never investigate the cause, so they never become aware that their implants are making them ill. He assured me there was no way to test that my implants were or were not causing my symptoms but that he would run a large panel of blood work to rule out any autoimmune disease my symptoms could be attributed to. I went through the motions of having my blood work done there in the office and waited patiently for the results...negative. My blood showed no autoimmune disease, which to me guaranteed that my ailments were my body's auto immune response to my 'perfectly safe lifetime devices'. These suspicions were confirmed when I looked further into the Facebook support groups and read countless stories of women who began getting ill just months or a few short years after getting implants but never associated their ailments to their implants. After living with illness for years, they then were diagnosed with full blow autoimmune diseases, many women seeing a reverse in symptoms and even bloodwork showing loss of autoimmune diagnosis after explant surgery. Although our symptoms varied from woman to woman, the one thing each of us women had in common was we were all told our implants were perfectly safe. Some of us women were even told that they were 'lifetime devices', never needing to be revised. There are heartbreaking stories of women who lived with implants and illness for 20, 30 plus years, and were now bed-ridden and not even strong enough to survive explant surgery. Stories of women who were now battling cancer caused by their implants. I cried a lot at my computer reading these devastating stories. I cried for myself and I cried for each of these women who were so sick, and just like me could no longer mother their children or be the person they used to be. I was also grateful for God guiding me to this information after only three short years of being ill. This in addition to all the stories of success after explant gave me hope for the future.

Just a few short days after seeing the rheumatologist, Matt and I were on our way to get the results of an ultrasound and CT scan that had been done for my throat. I was now having pain in my throat and difficulty swallowing along with severe reflux.

"Your bloodwork looks great," Doc Alex said to me. "So, you're feeling well," he continued with more of a statement than a question. I could feel my heart pounding inside me, as I looked around the room wondering if Matt or the doctor could hear it, it seemed that loud to me. My eyes began to tear up and I said, "I don't feel well at all, Doc, I am dying of something. I think it's my breast implants that are making me sick." To my surprise he didn't look at me crooked or even tell me I was crazy. He turned toward me, looked up from his laptop for what seemed like the first time ever, met my eyes and replied, "I think you could be right." I had to refrain from jumping off the exam table to hug him! I felt a wave of relief rush through me, having just been validated by the man who has been sending me for so many tests to help me figure out what was wrong. Matt was quiet but he perked up to attention to hear what the doctor had to say. We listened as the doctor explained that breast implants are foreign objects; our body recognizes that and attempts to fight them off. This response from our body can create a storm inside of us and our immune system goes into overdrive in attempt to rid itself of these objects. This immune response, as well as the toxins and heavy metals we are exposed to, will create illness. I thanked the doctor for believing me and I cried, having felt a sense of hope for the first time in a long time. What Doc Alex had said made sense to me about my immune system working so hard to protect me from these implants. I was lucky, I thought to myself. Having heard all those heartbreaking stories in my support group of women who had been ill for years and never connecting the dots, until they had full-blown autoimmune diseases. Diseases that could be better managed after the removal of implants, but would always be present in their bodies. I knew at that moment; this was the ember inside me. The burning deep within that had taken my life as I once knew it and turned it upside down.

"What are my options, Doc?" I asked. He said, "I have tested you for everything and all your tests come back normal. At this point your options are to keep your implants and be sick, or take them out and hope that's the answer to your problems." Feeling that this was quite a leap of faith, to have surgery without knowing if it will help, Matt and I drove home quiet and numb.

I didn't dream that night. There was no digging, no swimming or running, nothing. When I awoke the next day I knew the meaning behind the dreams I had been having for the weeks that led me to this imperative information. A higher power was sending signs through my unconscious, guiding me to keep digging for the information I needed to change my life. I couldn't keep living like this. I wasn't living. This was no life I wanted to have. I would have never thought that my 'perfectly safe lifetime devices' could make me so ill. This is a side effect you would expect to see or hear about before agreeing to a major surgery like a breast augmentation. After three years of illness I was all too familiar with side effects of medications and procedures. Even my children at their young age are conscious of the dreadful list of things that can happen from some medicines just by watching TV commercials. So how in the world, if breast implants are made of toxic chemicals that at times require a biohazard bag after removal, did I never hear about one side effect prior to my digging for information? I was lied to. We were all lied to.

I am a woman of action, and I needed a plan. As I processed all this devastating information about the heavy metals released by both silicone and saline implants and the autoimmune reaction they cause, I continued to research. These support groups became my home. A place I could go to feel understood and never judged. This was a priceless gift to me at this point to assist me through the stages of healing I was about to embark upon. I made an appointment with my plastic surgeon. I needed to speak to him about my desire to have these toxic bags taken out of me. The pace I was moving came as a bit of a shock to Matt, but he agreed to come with me to the appointment for support. "It's like a splinter," I said to Matt. You get a splinter in your finger, your body knows it doesn't belong there. It hurts, it becomes red, swollen and irritated. Sometimes causing pain to the entire finger. If left long enough, you risk infection and other ailments. So what do you do? You get it out, ASAP, by any means necessary because it's not supposed to be there.

"What if you have your implants out and you don't get any better?" a friend asked me. My response came easy. I told her that every ounce of my being was telling me this was my issue. Feeling toxic and sick was my incredible body's way of telling me something was very wrong. I explained that I was

82

confident explant surgery was the right decision for me. Even if my symptoms didn't improve, my textured implants were putting me at risk for Breast Implant Associated Lymphoma. Had I known my chances of cancer would increase due to implants, I never would have gotten them. "So," I said to my friend, "If there is any chance of me saving myself and getting my life back, explant is where it begins." I explained that the moment I realized my beautiful breast implants were the cause of the fire inside me, I wanted them out. I wanted them out now! I no longer cared that they were beautiful. All I saw when I looked in the mirror were 'foreign objects' that were toxic inside me, trying to take my life. All I knew was that they were not going to win.

Chapter Seven

~Forgive Me Father For I Knew Not What I Was Doing...~

Sometimes the only way to truly grow in faith is to walk through a time in your life when your faith is constantly tested. These past few months had certainly made me lose faith in doctors after being bounced around from "ologist" to "ologist" with no answers. However, day-by-day I could feel a pull inside me, a voice if you will. I strongly felt God was beside me; gently guiding me forward, not letting me give in like I wanted to. I was tired...so tired of feeling sick and tired that I got on my knees and prayed. I prayed so hard. I prayed that God would hold my hand and help me figure out what was wrong with me. "Why didn't you ever give up?" my mom said to me one day. "What made you keep searching for answers?" she asked. "It was God, Mom," I replied. He was there with me through it all. I just hadn't seen it until my weakest point. Once my eyes were opened, he was everywhere and the signs were glorious. Having my eyes opened to this gave me a whole new perspective on life.

Although I was beyond tired at this point, I made it a priority to get to Church each week I was able. Maddie would usually join me on Sunday mornings. Watching her watch me gently sob through each sermon broke my heart. I still hadn't had the heart to tell her just how sick I was feeling; however, to some extent, she knew without me saying. That is the strangest part of illness caused by breast implants. Most of us women look perfectly normal on the outside. Aside from the tired eyes or hint of sickness in our coloring, we look pretty healthy. For me, it was the face full of painful acne that also gave it away. So when I would come undone during worship, Maddie would silently excuse herself from the pew and retrieve tissues for me to dry my eyes. In those weeks I wasn't just hearing the sermon from the pastor, I was *feeling* the words that were so eloquently spoken. It was as if the words were written just for me each week. I was continuously amazed at the messages I was receiving. I distinctly remember the sermon that was given the week before I met with my plastic surgeon to discuss explant surgery. My pastor spoke of Jesus on the cross. As his beaten body hung from the cross, growing weaker and weaker, Jesus spoke; "Forgive them Father for they know not what they do". Those words rang in my head that week.

The moment I sat across from my plastic surgeon looking at me with doubt in his eyes about the sickness I was experiencing, I heard those words. As the surgeon looked me in the eyes, he justified every ailment I was having. He ended the appointment with the bold statement of, "I could take your implants out for you if you want. Every woman is entitled to change her mind." Every ounce of me wanted to scream! However, I didn't. I calmly replied, "This is not about me changing my mind, this is about me wanting my health and my life back." I focused on forgiveness that day as I walked out of his office; not making a six-month appointment for the first time, not making any appointment for that matter. I just collected my things and myself and I left.

For days after, I prayed for forgiveness for my surgeon. I forgave him, for he knows not what he does. This message came to me at just the right time. To this day I only pray that someday he will see the truth. I pray he and the other surgeons recognize that Breast Implant Illness is real and women deserve to be fully informed before deciding to implant. I continued to think of this message in the days, weeks, and even now still when I stumble upon a negative comment with regard to my situation. A hurtful encounter is much more tolerable when it's met with forgiveness. I came to realize I also needed to forgive myself. Forgiveness for the decision I made to get implants. Forgiving myself for believing I wasn't enough just as God made me. Forgiving yourself seems to be a greater feat than offering the forgiveness of others. It's a process and I am trusting in God that I will get there in His time. I came to realize that had I known differently, I would have made wiser choices. I needed to forgive myself for I knew not what I was doing.

At 38 years old, I finally learned how to pray. The funny thing about praying is that it's just like Googling. When you Google information on the Internet, you've got to know the right questions to ask in order to get the information you desire. When you pray, you have to be mindful of what to pray for. All my life I prayed that I would do well on a test or I prayed that I would get the job I wanted or I'd pray my annual pap test would come back negative. I would even pray the purse I'd been eyeing up would go on sale!

These past few months I had been praying that I wouldn't die from whatever was making me ill. Yet another sermon came my way and I learned that I was praying all wrong. I wasn't inputting the correct prayers into my internal Google search bar. The pastor spoke about how we are not to ask God for health and good fortune but rather to ask him to be with us and guide us along whatever path he has chosen for us. So, I began to do just that, I didn't pray for God to keep me alive or for my health to be that of perfection... I simply told God 'whatever will be will be, just be near me.' This trust I now had in God had given me the tools I needed to continue moving forward toward health and healing. I was armed with a strong faith that I knew would serve me well along my journey.

My journey continued after the disappointing meeting with my plastic surgeon. Just because he didn't believe my illness was due to my breast implants didn't mean I was going to give up. That's when God sent me Dr. Buinewicz. I found a support group that was local to my area and many women were raving about Doc B. He was an experienced plastic surgeon of many years that had recently begun to help many women suffering with Breast Implant Illness get the proper explant to heal. It seemed like a lifetime waiting for my consult with him; each day feeling like I was growing sicker and sicker.

Just before consultation day, I received a call from my Functional Medicine Nurse Practitioner, Elaine. You see, long before learning about Breast Implant Illness, I felt frustrated by medical practices that wanted to just treat my symptoms, rather than address what could be causing them. It was then that I found Elaine. She saw the desperation in my eyes a year earlier when we met and I sobbed over how uncomfortable my acne was and how anxious and depressed I was feeling.

Elaine told me she was inspired by my mission to figure out what was ailing me and in turn she worked tirelessly to help me. Over the past year I had tested positive for SIBO (small intestine bacterial overgrowth). This is an intestinal disease that results in the inability of the body to absorb nutrients from the intestine and may lead to malnutrition and vitamin deficiencies. It causes indigestion, diarrhea, bloating, and abdominal pain, all of which I had. Having been treated for this by Elaine with two rounds of antibiotics in the past, I was still suffering. So after many supplements without relief, she ran a stool test. Boy, was that a real treat, to collect my sample at 6am on a Monday morning.

As I was driving home from work just two days before my consult with Dr. B, Elaine called with the results of my stool test. "Hey," she said, "I have your results." I listened intently as I pulled my car into a lot so I could concentrate. "Let me ask you this," she began. "Do you have diarrhea all day, every day?" she asked. Finding her question kind of funny, I giggled a little. "Not all day," I replied. But now that I was thinking about it, I never really did have a normal poop either. As I told her this, she confirmed that made sense according to the results of my stool test. "You have h-pylori and a ton of parasites in your stool, your gut is really sick," she told me. "What is going on with you, Tara?" she asked. I hadn't had the chance to see her in a while and things had been moving so fast that she was unaware of all the research I had been doing and my thoughts of Breast Implant Illness.

I threw my head in my hands and began to sob right there on the side of the road in my car with Elaine on the other end of the phone. She gave me a moment, and as I composed myself I said, "I think I know what's wrong with me, Elaine, I think my breast implants are making me sick." She was silent just for a brief moment when she responded with, "That would make a lot of sense." Validation! Again! I cried harder at the thought that I knew I was on the right track, but to hear her confirm it, along with Doc Alex, made me so grateful. She listened as I filled her in on the research I had done and the support group I discovered. Before she hung up with me that day she told me how proud she was of me for discovering what could possibly be the cause of all these symptoms I'd been having. Of all the emotions I had felt over these past few months, proud wasn't one I had felt. After we hung up, I continued to cry but her words hung in my head. Proud was something I needed to feel. I wasn't there yet but until she said it, I wasn't even aware that proud was something I *should* be feeling. After all, I was only trying to save my life. For me, this was just survival.

When consultation day with Dr. Buinewicz finally arrived, I was nervous, however, I was armed with a list of questions gathered and recommended by our support group. The doctor and his nurse entered the room gently. I knew he had read my medical files I left with his office staff. He came in and said, "Well, you have a very interesting story." He sat next to me as I told him about getting my textured silicone 'gummy bear' implants in 2015 and after only a month my lymph nodes swelled in my armpits. I told him about the fatigue, frequent urination, panic attacks, heart palpitations, pain, difficulty breathing, food sensitivities, joint pain, brain fog, low libido,

h-pylori, parasites, depression, vision issues, and of course I didn't have to tell him about the acne-that he could see the moment he entered the room. He listened graciously as I cried just thinking about all these symptoms that crept up slowly over time but led me to feel as though I was dying. I cried thinking, *Here I am taking a huge leap of faith hoping that a major surgery that will take my beautiful breasts away will help my illness.* This ugly illness that no one could really see but I was aware it existed every moment of every day. I cried because no one told me any of these symptoms were a possibility of these 'safe lifetime devices'. I didn't want to have surgery again! I was sad and Doc B was patient as I cried. He chuckled as my husband joked that crying is what I was best at these days. "Don't worry, Doc, it'll pass, just give her a minute," Matt joked.

Doc B explained the entire surgery to us and did a thorough exam. Just by palpating my left breast, he could pinpoint where my pain had been for the past year without me saying a word. He sat and explained to Matt and I about the capsule that your body begins to form the moment the breast implants are placed. Your body recognizes these foreign objects and begins to attempt to protect itself by forming tissue around the implant. Doc B explained, this capsule would have to be removed for me to fully heal from the illness I was experiencing. The compassion and understanding of Breast Implant Illness Dr. B showed me was the reason I left knowing he would be the surgeon to take my implants out. My prayers were being answered. I had found three trusted doctors that believed in Breast Implant Illness and supported my decision to remove my implants. Although I didn't need their approval, I had prayed for strength to move forward toward healing and this is just what I needed. My prayers were being answered and I was ready to take this leap of faith.

Chapter Eight

~ Tata to Tara's Toxic Tits ~

Just a few short weeks passed between my consultation with Dr. B and my explant surgery date. May 4th was eviction day for these toxic bags of shit, and I was nervous and excited all at the same time. At this point I wasn't keeping anything a secret anymore. People at work knew I was sick. They watched during the past months as I struggled to get through the day, or I was absent all the time due to doctors' appointments and tests. By now, I had gone through an MRI of my breasts and hip, CT scan of my throat, ultrasound of my carotid arteries, a chest x-ray, a stress test, and an echocardiogram, as well as tons of bloodwork. It's amazing I hadn't turned into a zombie after all the radiation and vials of blood taken from me. Although, zombie would explain how I looked and felt at that point.

A week before my surgery I was a bundle of nerves. Having felt so very sick for so long I was unsure if my body would handle a major surgery well. To be very honest, I spent most days trying to talk myself down about thoughts of dying during surgery. I knew that Matt was aware of my wishes for if I died, because it was a talk we had earlier in the year before I gained the knowledge about Breast Implant Illness. "I'm dying, I would say to him," as he would hold me while I sobbed in his arms. I told him my wishes for myself and for him, and of course I had a whole plan of how he could raise the girls without me. He listened but was quiet about it. I am not sure he knew how to respond, or if there was even a right way to respond. He just listened and that was best. As I attempted to remain calm and stop envisioning what my family's life would look like if this surgery killed me, I knew in that last week I needed to find peace. Peace in my heart that whatever was meant to happen, would, and that I would have God to hold my hand the entire time.

I reached out to my Pastor. I emailed him my story from beginning to end, with all the horror in the middle. He called me, exactly a week before "B" day. He listened as I reiterated the stories of how I came to believe God was guiding me along my journey, and he was thrilled to learn I'd been a witness to this level of faith. He prayed with me and for me. He prayed for my surgeon and the nurses that would be with me that next week. I cried. The peace I needed had found me in his final words, "All will be well." Those words remained close in my heart that following week leading up to surgery. Any moment I found myself drowning into that dark space, I would say those words over and over again in my head. All will be well. I had come to learn that those words didn't mean that there was any guarantee that I would come out of surgery healed. I learned that those words were the only guarantee God could provide to any of us. That no matter what the storm brings, the promise is that you will never be alone. If I were to have this surgery and my worst fear came true, I had the promise my family would be ok. If I were to have the surgery and was not healed of my illness, I wouldn't be alone then, either. With this peace came strength and with the strength came the confidence I needed to know I was doing the right thing. Taking this leap of faith was exactly where I was meant to be. The days following my conversation with my pastor, I spent my time envisioning myself waking up, bright eyed and healthy from surgery. Each time the anxiety would attempt to overtake me, I would close my eyes and see myself living again. I would envision spending quality time with family and friends. I pictured what it would look like to have my life back and the visions were so vivid I could almost feel it!

May 4, 2018, I awoke early from a deep sleep. It was a glorious spring day, and Matt and I packed up the car to drive the hour and a half to the surgery center. I felt good. I felt ready! Feeling so good in fact, the medication Doc B prescribed to keep me calm before surgery was unnecessary. My mind and my body were filled with such a sense of peace and calm; I was in awe. Matt and I enjoyed our drive together, hand in hand, talking and laughing and enjoying the beautiful scenery of the Pennsylvania back roads. "You doing OK?" Matt would ask. "I am more than OK, Love," I responded. I wasn't lying, all things seemed as though they had fallen into place and I was right where I was meant to be.

The sense of calm remained with me as we arrived at the surgery center. As I checked in, I was greeted by so many wonderful nurses and an anesthesiologist who put me at ease. He sat down and listened to my concerns. I shared with him

97

how coming out of anesthesia with my augmentation took days. I was out of it for a long time and in so much pain. He assured me he wouldn't let that happen to me and I trusted him. I kissed Matt goodbye on my way down the hall, dressed in the ever-flattering gown, hair net and non-slip socks. I was assisted onto the OR table and like little worker bees the nurses started hooking things up and taking blood pressures. The nurse at my feet was confirming my information: name, birthday, the usual. "What procedure are you here for today?" she asked. "To get these toxic bags of shit out of me," I responded with some sass. All the nurses laughed and I followed up with, "Although it's probably written down as an explant with total capsulectomy."

Before long, Doc B and my anesthesiologist entered the room and immediately began to help me fall asleep. "Do you feel anything?" the doctor asked. I told him I did. My arm and throat began to feel cold and numb. He told me that was the anesthesia beginning to work. "It tastes like shit," were my last words to him and he chuckled. Then, he squeezed my hand as he told me not to worry. He would take good care of me. My last thought as I closed my eyes was 'all will be well'.

Beep—beep—beep, *what's that noise*, I thought as I attempted to open my eyes. Beep—beep—beep, it's the heart monitor, that's the beat of my heart. I'M ALIVE!!!! A single tear ran down my cheek as I opened my eyes to see the grateful sight of the recovery room. I had never felt such relief in my whole life. All of a sudden, the worrying and planning for my demise seemed so far behind me. I had an overwhelming feeling of gratitude to just be awake, and for the first time in a very long time, I felt truly alive. *Must be the drugs,* I thought to myself. Unable to focus on the clock to check the time, or even remember the time I entered the operating room, I just gave a quiet, "Hello?" I was greeted by a kind nurse who said my heart rate was slightly elevated but was coming down and I did great. I asked for my husband and thought back to my last surgery. I wasn't moaning or crying for Matt this time. This surgery was already feeling very different from the implant surgery. Matt came to me and he told me Doc B said the surgery went great, and although he had to work very diligently to get the entire capsule out, he was successful. It is imperative that the surgeon removes the entire capsule during explant surgery. The capsule is tissue that your body forms in attempt to protect you from your breast implants. With both silicone and saline implants, the chemicals that make up the outer shell begin to leach into your body. The materials that implants are made of are not meant to survive inside a body that is 98 degrees or warmer. These chemicals leach through the capsule that surrounds the implant and infiltrates the bloodstream. This process then creates the storm of possible symptoms that many women experience. To hear that Doc B was able to rid my body of my capsules was music to my ears. He also informed Matt that I had a fair amount of Biofilm inside my chest wall. Later, he explained to us that biofilms are another way the body works to fight a foreign object. It's like a chronic infection triggered by the inflammation and it "looked like green snot," as Dr. B told us. Biofilm is known to create *P. acnes* and *staph infection*, both of which were detected on my face by my dermatologist. "I am curious to see how your skin heals after your surgery," Dr. B said to me.

Unlike my last experience, within minutes I was talking, calling my mom and getting dressed. There was pain but it was a manageable pain, and I was ALIVE so I didn't give a crap about the pain anyway. Pain is only temporary and I was so grateful to be alive and out of surgery.

We needed to stay the night in a local hotel as precaution for the first 24 hours. While Matt and I sat in the hotel room binge watching Netflix and eating Italian takeout, I kept mentally preparing myself for the pain that would come after the nerve block wore off. I waited, and waited and the pain never came. I kept reflecting on three years prior when I had my implants put in and I felt so awful for days and days. I was now coming to realize that my breast implants began sucking the life out of me from day one. "There is more life in you just hours after surgery, than there has been in the last 3 years," Matt said to me as I sat across from him eating my ravioli and planning what I wanted to do over the summer. I just smiled at him and relished in the overwhelming feeling of gratitude I had. I was grateful that the surgery went well, grateful I woke up from the surgery and grateful that within hours I knew this leap of faith had changed my life for the better.

Early the next morning, I spoke with Dr. B and assured him I was feeling fine. He gave me the 'all clear' to go home. As we drove home that day, I was elated and prayed it wasn't just the effects of the anesthesia and the IV fluids I received the day before. Most of the car ride home was quiet as Matt and I both enjoyed the silent time to reflect. I turned to him and said "Thank you." Without giving him time to question me, I continued, "Thank you for all you have done for me to help me get through this time. Thank you for all the times you just let me cry and tell you how scared I was, even

101

though I know you were scared yourself." He squeezed my hand and responded with, "I love you, Tara, and I just want you to be healthy so we can grow old together." For the remainder of the time it took to get home I just grew further and further into a space of such gratitude. My thoughts drifted to my mother, who listened to me complain about the lack of answers from doctors, cry about being sick, and sob about being so scared. I know that she too was scared. I was grateful for both Matt and my mom! They were my rocks through those months. I was grateful for friends who supported me at my darkest moments while away from home. I was grateful for Maddie and Lexie and the unconditional love they showed me because I hadn't been the mother they needed in a long while. In my darkest days, there were times my daughters assumed the role of adult and stepped in when I was too weak or too ill. I also had an overwhelming feeling of gratitude for Doc B. I was feeling so grateful for his gentle spirit, his true belief in Breast Implant Illness, and his skills as a surgeon. He was the man who had just given me my life back; he was a true hero to me.

This feeling of gratitude stays with me, even today. Life doesn't promise to be easy, but it's full of lessons that help us evolve. We must allow ourselves to be open to these lessons to grow and move forward in our lives; become stronger, better people. Once your health is taken from you, life has a way of putting things into perspective. Gratitude is a gift.

Chapter Nine

~ The Heal is Real ~

The road to full recovery is like driving full speed down Lombard Street in San Francisco. There are twists and turns that come on sudden and sharp and sometimes you've got to hold on for dear life. The first week after surgery was better than expected. Matt was my nurse those first few days, helping me use the bathroom and empty my drains. I needed assistance on/off the couch because although there was minimal pain, it was worse if I did too much moving around. The risk of bleeding is greater with a total capsulectomy compared to a breast augmentation. The reason for this is because the surgeon has to remove the entire capsule out of you. The capsule is the scar tissue that forms around the implant immediately upon implantation. Scar capsule is your body's immune response to the foreign objects and often grows beyond the implants into the armpits and ribs, often close to the lungs. This leaves your chest area vulnerable to excess bleeding, called a hematoma. Hematomas are a risk with any surgery and with any surgeon. In our support group we've watched some women require second surgeries to stop the bleeding in the days after explant.

I worked very hard to keep my new found energy at bay and rest as much as I could. Rest is key in the first days after explant. Keeping your arms down at your sides and moving at a minimum to assure you recover well and keep bleeding and swelling to a minimum. The couch was my home base in these days, and eventually Matt had showed Lexie how to empty my drains. The girls enjoyed being a part of my recovery process. Taking care of someone who can't care for themselves is a great learning experience and one they embraced. I only had my drains for 4 days, and although it felt weird to have them taken out, I was thankful to be free of them. By day six I was in desperate need of a shower and I was healed enough to help myself. It wasn't pretty, but I got the job done. Aside from the general fatigue of just having surgery, my recovery was going better than I could have hoped for.

I just kept thinking back to my augmentation surgery, and how difficult it was for me to recover from that. Looking back, it's almost as if my body never did recover from getting the implants, because I was truly never the same afterward. The symptoms come on so slowly over time that it's almost as if you can miss them. You justify in your head how they could be caused from being busy with everyday life, or maybe just at 'the age' where your body is beginning to 'change'. Until you reach the point when the illness becomes too severe to justify anything anymore. I stayed out of work for two weeks after explant surgery. I enjoyed some time with family and friends who came to visit and rested as much as possible. Dr. B kept a close eye on me, and I was grateful because he was available by cell at any time. The week prior to surgery, I spent a lot of time envisioning what being healed would look and feel like for me. I truly believe that keeping my mind in this positive, forward thinking space aided in my recovery. Never once did I need to call the doctor or even take any pain medicine. I was in constant awe of how much different this recovery was than the last one. My body knew immediately what my mind took three years to discover: my breast implants had made me deathly ill.

After surgery, the immediate change in me was my energy level. I began to wake up feeling rested for the first time in a very long time. I was finding that I was able to work my full 40-hour a week schedule and even come home and do the never ending 'running around' with the kids after work. By month two-post op I noticed I could stay up until 10:30-11:00 some nights, which was late for me by my recent standards. My newfound energy meant I was more productive and able to really be present for my family! Since explant, I have not once woken up from a deep sleep in a full-blown panic attack and my depression has lifted. My vision that was constantly blurry before has cleared and I no longer feel as though I am drunk all the time. If you have not experienced Breast Implant Illness, this may sound crazy but it's like living in a fog every day. The memory loss subsided during the first three months of recovery, and my lost libido was found! Hallelujah! No longer feeling dead on the inside has been the most exciting thing to happen post explant. The constant pain I had in my throat and the silent reflux has gone away, as did the need to urinate all the time. It's almost as if I can hear my kidneys thanking me for no longer having to work overtime to flush out all those toxins running through my body. I no longer have difficulty catching my breath, or feel like an elephant is sitting on my chest. The restless legs, heart palpitations, the perpetual itchy skin and food sensitivities have disappeared.

Slowly but surely, I am becoming the 'who' I once was, and it feels amazing. Some symptoms of my illness have been slower to return to normal, like the constant ringing in my ears, irregular periods, hair loss, and my acne. The important thing is that my acne is improving every day and regardless of my small breakouts now, I am 100% more comfortable and no longer need ice packs on my face for pain.

Although the 'heal is real,' flare-ups are a fact of healing from Breast Implant Illness that we have to live through. The inflammation that your body had been fighting, returns, with a vengeance. Like a true ember, that inflammation can radiate a substantial amount of heat long after the fire has been extinguished. When a flare up happens, you go from feeling on top of the world, having your life back, to having the rug swept out from under your feet. I will wake up one morning, and suddenly feel anxious and depressed again. The fatigue overtakes my body, my throat aches, and my acne rears its ugly head and reminds me just how difficult it is to suffer from teenage acne at almost 40.

My lymph nodes have gotten smaller, but during flare-ups these lymph nodes become large and sore all over again. These flare-ups are frustrating, and I am trying to trust in God and His process that all things will eventually return to normal and stay that way for good.

My worry is always that all these symptoms will never disappear again. They do though. For me, they stay for about a week or two and then just as quickly as they come on, they disappear. I am lucky though, flare-ups last longer for many women. Our warrior sisters say they live through these types of flare-ups for about a year or more before they completely subside, although healing looks different for everyone. For any of my fellow warrior sisters living through healing, remember to treat your bodies with respect and love. Flare-ups will happen. Try to utilize clean, healthy organic foods to keep the fire inside extinguished. If your body is not cared for properly, you can rekindle the fire within you. Just stay calm, honor those feelings during your flares. Let them strengthen you by reflecting on how far you've come in your healing journey.

The most difficult part of healing actually has nothing to do with the physical aspects of heath. The emotional journey Breast Implant Illness survivors go through is the piece of the puzzle that keeps us from feeling whole. Women choose to get breast implants for various reasons. Those who decided to get breast implants to enhance their look, or those who get them for reconstruction because they were survivors of breast cancer. There are women with uneven breasts who get implants to balance out their chest. Some women, like in my case, are very small chested and decide that implants will give them a larger chest in order to look more feminine. Other women are well endowed, but are led to believe that getting implants to become even bigger breasted will somehow help them gain more confidence. Then there are our double warrior sisters who had been dealt the card of breast cancer. No matter what the reason for getting their implants, all women are led by society to believe that a life without large perky breasts is somehow inadequate; somehow *we* are inadequate. So whatever the reason that leads a woman to get her implants, when she comes to the realization that they are what is making her ill; it's devastating.

The first devastation is realizing that you chose to subject your body to these foreign objects, or that you were lied to and made to believe you had no other options. Either way, in order to regain your health and save your own life, you must now reverse this decision. The second devastation is facing our reasoning for getting breast implants in the first place, head on. You are haunted by all the reasons you had self-esteem low enough to make you believe that you were not enough, just as God made you. If you had gotten your implants for reconstruction, you face the harsh reality that not only did your real breasts try to kill you, but so did your fake ones.

Some, if not all, plastic surgeons make you sign an informed consent prior to explant that makes you aware of just how emotionally devastating it can be to delete your boobs from your equation. I initialed next to statements like: I am aware that explant can create marital issues, I am aware that explant can play a negative role in my self-esteem, I am aware that the loss of my implants can possibly make me deformed. Imagine being sick and desperate enough to agree that the possible loss of your marriage, your self-esteem and the risk of deformity is better than the alternative. The alternative being a life trapped inside a toxic body that forces you to just exist, rather than truly live. It's not enough that we have to make this 'live or die a slow death' decision, but to also have to trudge through the emotional swamp on our way to health. It is draining. For me personally, I promised myself the moment I learned about Breast Implant Illness that I would love my body after explant regardless of what anyone said.

It has been difficult not to focus on the fact that things could have been very different for me, if only I had more information upon deciding to get breast implants. I have made a promise to myself, and our community. I will forever advocate for Breast Implant Illness. Upon breast augmentation surgery, there needs to be information shared that there is a possibility your implants could make you ill. Women should be given the knowledge that implants can cause a negative auto immune reaction, as well as various other health issues. Regardless if there is a rupture or your implants remain intact. Regardless if your implants are silicone or saline, they all begin to leach inside and expose our precious bodies to deadly chemicals. If one person told me that my textured implants put me at an increased risk for cancer, I would not have chosen to take that risk. Textured implants should not be used inside any woman, exposing them to such a risk. I have let go of the anger for not being more informed. I believe God has walked me through this journey to help spread the word, and allow women to be more informed. We deserve that much.

At nine months' post-surgery, I can honestly say I have remained committed to educating others, advocating, and learning to truly love my body and myself. There are women however, who will suffer from extended depression due to the loss of their implants. Marriages struggle and suffer because of the way our American society worships big boobs. This emotional rollercoaster is the toughest part of the healing because women are constantly being led to believe that we are not enough according to a society where 'enough' is only achieved by such extreme measures.

The men in our lives are also on a healing journey of their own and we need to be mindful of this. I've learned though our support groups that some women healing from BII had implants before they met their significant others. Some women got implants after they met their mate, and some got implants because of their significant others. Whatever the case, I believe each man will go through his own process. For me, Matt and I were together for many years before I chose to get implants. My implants seemed to balance out my figure, and he had no complaints about that. He grew attached to me having them and he enjoyed them being around. After explant, he was torn somewhere between wanting me to be healthy and losing his *breast friends*. He was angry that we had both been led to believe the implants were completely safe, and I would have them for the rest of my life. There was an anger that we both shared in the fact that I had chosen to get them at all. A serious regret we both had to work through. I escaped the feeling of loss when I removed my implants because for me, feeling alive again was so much greater than any feeling of loss. So, although the heal is real...it is also really difficult.

Chapter Ten

~ This IS Your Perfect~

It was when I was strong enough to get back to the gym that I realized everything had changed for me. Getting back to the gym after surgery was a surreal experience. My mind felt I had belonged there all along, but my body was torn and tired. I was welcomed with open arms and cried with members who were inspired by my story. While working out, things felt the same yet everything was different. I was starting over, lifting weights so light that I would almost chuckle to myself. It was a humbling experience for me to workout alongside girls who I had trained during the one year I worked as a personal trainer prior to my implants. Watching them throw weights around like I used to, some days I laughed about it and other days I cried. Some days I even cried in the middle of a set, dumbbells in hand and the tears would just overwhelm me. Most days though, I was proud. So proud of how far I had come. Like Elaine said, I was proud that I never gave up on discovering what was wrong with me. We must be our own advocates. I grew to realize I was beginning to embrace my story, my journey, and my storm that had brought me to who I am meant to be. The gift I was getting was the ability to love me just as God made me. With all my scars and all my flaws, I was truly learning to love myself. Exercise was no longer about what I looked like, it was slowly becoming about being the healthiest, happiest me I could be. My eyes no longer lingered at the mirrors and when I did catch a glimpse of myself I found I was no longer beating myself up for what I felt was inadequate. I was soaking up every bit of feeling proud of what I had and how far I had come, after almost losing it all.

My acne saved my life! If anyone understands looking in the mirror and not liking what you see, it's me. For years that seemed like forever, I had severe acne all over my face. I lived through cruel comments about how I looked and questions as to why my face looked so bad. The acne got so bad that makeup wasn't even an option anymore so I stopped hiding behind it. Although the pain in my face was constant, I would muster up the courage to go out in public and pretend the acne wasn't there. It was, however, very much there. Every time I looked in the mirror I was reminded that I looked different than everyone else. At times I would be eating, and my face would bleed from a blemish around my mouth. Still today, I have scars on my face and active breakouts that are nothing like what they used to be, but these imperfections have become a part of me. I have learned to change my way of thinking around these issues. Had I not been reminded by the mirror every day that something wasn't right, I may not have worked so tirelessly to figure out what was wrong with me so soon.

It was because of those ugly bumps on my face that I started working with Elaine. Initially, we thought it was the acne that was creating the depression and anxiety. Today, we know better. It was the toxins running through my bloodstream that made me feel in constant fight or flight mode. It was the biofilm inside my body creating the awful acne. That awful acne motivated me to begin my research early on in my illness and therefore I believe I was led to healing earlier than most. The same biofilm that caused the acne could have possibly led me to a diagnosis of BIA-ALCL as well. So I must be thankful for each step of this journey. My acne saved my life for sure!

I am learning to become thankful for my scars for they tell my story. The scars that sit under my small saggy breasts make me proud. I have stopped being angry with myself for getting my implants. I made that choice as a young woman who believed a particular body part would create happiness. Those tight red scars beneath my chest belong to a much different person. This scarred woman is now defined by the beauty that resides within her. My beauty is seen through my ability to be a strong role model for my girls, managing a family full of challenges. My beauty can be witnessed by my loyal friendships and my ability to make people feel loved. My beauty shines through the way I can inspire people with my encouraging words. My beauty is seen through my inner strength. A good friend recently reminded me that my strong will to stay and fight through any situation makes me a beautiful warrior. These are the beauties that define me as a person.

We are all filled with our own definition of beauty. We just need to be aware of what it is and share it with the world.

Once we embrace our beauty, we then need to be bold enough not to let society define our existence. We must always be kind and speak kindly to our bodies and ourselves.

If anyone understands verbally accosting yourself, it's me. I have a Master's Degree in it. So get up, ladies, get up right now and find a mirror, any mirror and go to it. I'm talking to everyone here no matter what your journey has been: implants or not. Go to your mirror and look at *your* perfect. It's the image that reflects back at you, this is *your* perfect, just as you are right now. We have all become so conditioned to belittle ourselves in the mirror that we almost feel silly looking at our reflections and complimenting ourselves. Who decided that treating ourselves with respect and love was a shameful thing? When did we decide to let others dictate what is best for our souls? Why have we decided the opinions of others have such power over us that we believe we are defined by any single body part?

They say our brains are designed to retain the negative comments we hear, and forget the positive. It takes five compliments to outweigh one negative statement. So, if we consistently pass by a mirror and pick ourselves apart for what's not 'up to par' according to society, we will eventually believe these negative statements to be true. Stop competing with one another! Accept your differences and embrace the beauty of others. Worship friendships and the gift of loyalty and commitment rather than material possessions and fake body parts. Skin is meant to sag, faces are supposed to wrinkle, and bodies are designed to grow bigger or smaller in certain areas. So let us reverse our way of thinking, break through society's standards, and learn to love ourselves. God designed us just as we are supposed to be, this, right here, right now is our perfect.

To my sisters who are healing from BII or any other situation that has knocked the wind out of you... Love, is the greatest gift you can bestow upon yourself. Self-love is NOT self-ish! You are not greedy for putting yourself first in this life. This healing process is a long, difficult road and you must surround yourself with people who lift your spirit and fill your soul with joy. You must be bold enough to stand up for yourself if you find anyone treating you unkindly. Along your way, you must be strong enough to let go of who or what doesn't serve you well. Breast Implant Illness may have broken you, but you are beautifully broken. Your brokenness is not the final outcome. Your outcome is the reward of who you get to become after the storm is over. The storm that you are walking through is a gift. Healing is what happens as you slowly un-wrap your gift and see what beauty has blossomed from your storm. Stay grateful for your story and how far you have come. Embrace the scars, both seen and un-seen. Focus on the beauty of the future. Let go of the anger for what has happened, for those dark moments have made you the warrior you are.

Some women are lucky enough to fully heal from Breast Implant Illness, and others may never fully recover. The one thing we all have in common is that none of us will ever be the same after what we have been through. You must be strong enough to allow the scars of your illness to change you for the better, otherwise the toxic implants and those who deceived us will win. After you are able to rid yourself of the toxic implants and detox from everything that was making you ill, you must also let go of the anger that you hold toward what happened. That anger is an extension of your implants, an emotional poison that will weigh you down.

Let that go and be grateful. Grateful for your journey, your story, your body that fought like a warrior and won the war. I had a teacher once tell me, "The best revenge is to live well."

Live well, my warrior sisters, live well!

I Woke Up One Day ~ by Tara Hopko

I woke up one day,
And thought to myself.
Wouldn't it be nice,
To have a top shelf.

I'd feel like a woman,
Wear a real size brassiere.
My husband and I,
Would hold them so dear.

So doc put em' in.
370 cc's.
Little did I know,
I'd be brought to my knees.

They were fun, at first,
I sure fill out a dress.
But I began to start feeling,
I am a bit of a mess.

First it's fatigue,
Then a lymph node would swell.
My eyes look so sick...
I wonder if anyone can tell?

"Your hair doesn't grow" ...
The hairdresser would say.
I hear, "Why in the world,
Does your face look that way?"

Pain burning, pain stabbing,
Constant ringing in my ears.
I've grown oh-so unsure,
I can handle all these fears.

Day after day aging,
In double time.
Ouch- that pain, in my hip
Maybe this could be Lyme?

Oh-hey there doc
I can't breathe well, I say.
He cocks his head to the side,
Maybe try yoga someday?

"You're nervous, you're anxious
You worry too much".
But I fear it's these bags,
Causing all this weird stuff.

Each night as I sit,
With my husband and cry.
All, I can say is,
I feel I might die!

So I woke up one day,
And I looked at myself.
I still have great boobs,
But where is my health?

The 'who' I once was,
Has disappeared awful quick.
My body and soul,
Are left feeling sick.

What's wrong with me Doc?
I broke down and cried.
"Your blood-work looks good"
But I feel dead inside.

So I woke up one day,
Being brought to my knees.
I prayed to the heavens,
Someone help me please!

Was then that I found,
Info Nicole had shown.
Thousands of women,
I'm not alone!

Breast Implant Illness,
It's real and it's true.
If only I'd known....
If only we knew.

But I woke up one day,
Now I know what to do.
To my body and mind,
I must stay true.

From this nightmare I'm living,
I want to wake up.
Even if that means,
I'll be an A cup.

These bags have to go,
I will take my life back,
What I'll do is explant,
It's my plan of attack.

It's then, that the heal
Will begin to take start.
My body, my mind,
My soul and my heart.

I'll surely be sad,
To not fill out a dress.
But peace I will have
To let go of this stress.

Then I'll wake up one day,
To my daughters I'll say.
Look in the mirror and love yourself, this way!

To myself I will turn,
And then I will say.
I'm grateful for you,
And that you woke up one day!

If you or someone you know have breast implants and are suffering from multiple unexplained symptoms listed below, you could have Breast Implant Illness:

- Chronic Fatigue
- Brain Fog/Memory Loss
- Joint and muscle pain
- Hair Loss
- Swollen Lymph nodes
- Inflammation
- Hypo/Hyper Thyroid symptoms
- Hypo/Hyper Adrenal symptoms
- Premature Aging
- Low Libido
- Dry Eyes, Decline in Vision
- Difficulty Swallowing/Choking/Reflux
- Leaky Gut, IBS and SIBO
- Food Intolerances
- Ear Ringing
- Skin Rashes/Acne
- Heart Palpitations/Changes in Heart Rate
- Anxiety/Depression/Panic Attacks
- Frequent Urination
- Symptoms or Diagnosis of Auto-immune diseases such as; Lyme's, Lupus, Hashimoto's, Rheumatoid Arthritis, MS, etc.

*Note: this is not a complete list of symptoms. For the complete list and extensive information on Breast Implant Illness please visit **healingbreastimplantillness.com**

BIA-ALCL-
Breast Implant Associated Anaplastic Large Cell Lymphoma

It is a unique type of lymphoma- cancer of the immune system that is not as rare as once suspected.

RISK factors:
You are at risk of developing BIA-ALCL if you have (or had) textured implants or implant expanders.

SYMPTOMS can include but are not limited to the following:

- An increase (swelling) in breast size
- Pain in or around the breast
- The development of a lump or lumps in or around the breast or under the armpit
- Swollen lymph nodes
- Itching or redness of the skin or near the breast
- Fluid around the implant seen on imaging such as ultrasound and/or MRI
- Fever
- Night sweats

For further information and the full list of symptoms please visit, **biaalcl.com**